# WELLNESS
## IN THE WOODS

**HIKING FOR HEALTH, HEALING & HAPPINESS**

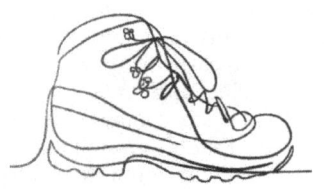

BY
DAVID HENTHORNE

Copyright © 2024 by David Henthorne

All rights reserved.

ISBN: 979-8-9909746-1-6

No portion of this book may be reproduced in any form without written permission from the publisher or author, except as permitted by U.S. copyright law.

This publication is designed to provide accurate and authoritative information in regard to the subject matter covered. It is sold with the understanding that neither the author nor the publisher is engaged in rendering legal, investment, accounting or other professional services. While the publisher and author have used their best efforts in preparing this book, they make no representations or warranties with respect to the accuracy or completeness of the contents of this book and specifically disclaim any implied warranties of merchantability or fitness for a particular purpose. No warranty may be created or extended by sales representatives or written sales materials. The advice and strategies contained herein may not be suitable for your situation. You should consult with a professional when appropriate. Neither the publisher nor the author shall be liable for any loss of profit or any other commercial damages, including but not limited to special, incidental, consequential, personal, or other damages.

Book cover and interior design by David Henthorne.

Cover photo by Hannah Henthorne.

Published by World of Wanders LLC
1st edition 2024

# Contents

| | |
|---|---|
| Thank you, boots | V |
| Introduction | VII |
| 1. Starting at the trailhead | 1 |
| 2. If we want more Father Time on our side, we need more Mother Nature | 9 |
| 3. Crooked trails help you think straight | 26 |
| 4. Let nature nurture your hurting heart | 35 |
| 5. More caring boot prints, less carbon footprint | 50 |
| 6. Taking the first steps | 59 |
| 7. Gear up for adventure! | 73 |
| 8. To all the trails I've loved before | 85 |
| 9. Happy trails to you | 119 |
| Acknowledgements | 126 |
| About the author | 128 |

# Thank you, boots

I owe my hiking boots a lot.

They've helped me through challenging times, on the trail and in life. Need some fresh air? Lace up the boots. Feeling stressed or depressed? Lace up the boots. Writer's block, creative lethargy, imagination on empty? Boot up.

They never complain that they're not "feeling it" today. They never talk back — even though they have tongues. They sit quietly in the closet or trunk of my car, waiting for their multi-mile moment in the sun. Whether I'm mourning a loss or just need a morning boost, they support me every step of the way.

My boots have propelled me, taking me up mountains, down canyons, and through forests to see the view from all perspectives. They've encouraged me to travel and explore different parts of the world I might not have considered before. They've motivated me professionally too, helping me craft a career and volunteer work that promotes tourism and the outdoors.

## DAVID HENTHORNE

And they inspired me to write this book. Kicked me in the butt you might say.

I've written a million ads and articles, jingles and jokes, posts and apologies, but I've never written a book — until now.

So thank you, boots. I couldn't do it without you.

# Introduction

*Even IYKYK, some things you might not know*

This book is an approachable approach to hiking for most people. I greatly admire those intrepid souls who challenge themselves with backpacking and through-hiking on long distance trails like the Pacific Crest Trail, the Appalachian Trail and others. But this isn't about that.

For this book we're defining "hiking" as an outdoor walk of three miles or more. A day hike. Mostly along natural terrain and unpaved trails where you're likely to encounter elevation changes, be they hills, foothills, mountains, or "Whoa, we gotta climb THAT?"

We're all busy and time-starved, and it can be difficult to carve out several hours on the trail plus the travel time to get there and back. For me an ideal hike is somewhere between 3-13 miles. A hike should feel more challenging than your average sidewalk stroll.

When does a "walk" become a "hike"? I'm not sure there's an official stance on this...but you know it when you feel it. Certainly there are health and wellness benefits of urban walks, suburban walks, treadmill walks, and anything cooked in a wok. But within these pages let's agree that hiking involves getting your heart rate up in the comforting embrace of nature. An exhilarating walk in the woods. A wonderful wander.

What are the wellness benefits of hiking? Well, there are plenty of them. It's more than mere physical health, although that's a big part of it. Wellness encompasses our physical, mental, emotional and spiritual health. While exercise and fitness get all the swole headlines, true well-being thrives on a deeper connection within ourselves and the world around us. And in my opinion, you won't find a better place to nourish that connection than the inviting embrace of a hiking trail.

## HIKING BENEFITS YOUR BODY, MIND + SOUL

As exhausting as a hike can sometimes be, I've never regretted a single one. I always get more out of it than I put in. Throughout these pages we'll explore the many life-changing, awe-inspiring, mood-boosting highs of hiking, and how hitting the trail can help so many people.

## WELLNESS IN THE WOODS

**Health benefits.** An outdoor hike is an ideal way to improve your physical and mental health — science says so. Fortunately it's also a low-impact activity that can be enjoyed by people of all ages and fitness levels. Hiking can help you hit specific health goals, from weight-loss to heart health to joint pain relief (my knees can vouch for this one).

**Connecting with nature.** Wander the woods and you're sure to find your inner naturalist, and gain a new appreciation for the beauty of your surroundings. This can help reduce stress, improve your mood, and boost your overall well-being. Nature is full of life and constantly healing itself. It can help you heal too.

**Learning about the environment.** Now more than ever, caring about our planet is essential. Earth needs our help. Trail hiking inspires you to learn more about the environment and the native plants and animals that live there. This can help you appreciate the natural world and understand the importance of protecting it. Yes, we all need to be Tree Huggers.

**Building relationships.** Hiking can certainly be enjoyed as a solo adventure. But a walk in the woods with your significant other, family, or group of friends is a powerful opportunity to bond with people you care about, get healthy, and share your love of nature.

# DAVID HENTHORNE

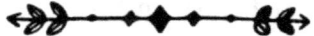

It took me quite some time to discover my love for trekking. In fact, I despised it growing up! I vividly remember post-dinner woods walks. As warm weather approached, we would head to a local Metro Park after dinner a few times per week. Spiders, an ornery blast of wind, and the rustling of leaves was enough to get me way worked up. That all changed the summer before I went off to college. We took a family trip to California, and half the trip we explored the majestic redwoods and panoramic vistas of Yosemite National Park. I felt like I was in a Disney movie. A friendly family of squirrels, misty waterfall kisses, the oh-so-satisfying ache in the legs back at our room in the lodge were my signs that hiking is a special thing.
– **Hannah, Colorado**

I've been walking the woods for as long as I can remember. My dad was an outdoorsman and would take me and my sister along. It sparked a life-long love of nature in both of us. – **Carie, Ohio**

# WELLNESS IN THE WOODS

I would say I started hiking on a regular basis when I moved to San Francisco in 1996. Hiking became a regular occurrence and an amazing way to learn about and enjoy the surroundings there.  **– John, Oregon**

## READY TO TAKE THE FIRST STEP?

While by no means a comprehensive guide, this book offers some simple tips and adventures from a happy hiker. Think of it as a "trail map" for getting started. Or at least how I did. Throughout these pages I'll share research I've rounded up, helpful Hike Hacks, and Top Trails that have stayed with me long after I knocked the mud off my boots. I've also asked fellow hiking enthusiasts I admire for their insights and inspiration.

I hope this book helps you choose the right gear, pick the right routes, blaze your own trail, get lost...and find yourself.

# Chapter 1

# Starting at the trailhead

*An oh-so-brief history of hiking*

So who started this whole hiking thing?

Traveling by foot is as old as mankind itself. Ever since our ancestors crawled out of the primordial soup, we've walked everywhere for food, safety, commerce and war. Walking was the way since we could walk upright and stopped all that knuckle dragging. But as far as who gets the credit for "inventing" hiking...all trails seem to lead to famed Italian poet and scholar Francesco Petrarca.

## The Father of Hiking

On April 26, 1336 Petrarca became the first person who claimed to climb a mountain just for the sake of the experience. He wrote about his ascent of Mont Ventoux, a 6,270-ft mountain in the Provence region of southern France, in a well-known letter to a friend. He says he was motivated purely by the desire to see the view from the top. Because of this, he has been called "the first tourist."

Petrarca (apparently better known as Petrarch) was more than just a mountaineer though. He has been called the "Father of Humanism" and even the "Father of the Renaissance" itself. He traveled widely throughout Europe and was an ambassador. His writing was used to shape the modern Italian language we know today. Look, the guy kept busy, ok.

He was an accomplished academic, a celebrity of the time, and would have been believed without question. And while modern scholars may differ on the accuracy of Petrarca's climbing claim, the case can be made that he can be called the "Father of Hiking."

## Such a Wanderful Word

So we have (supposedly) the first hike. What about the origin of the word itself?

While its exact provenance is not 100% known, the word "hike" winds its way back to a couple centuries ago. According to etymologists (AKA "word nerds"), the earliest version of hike seems to be "yike," a word from 1736 meaning "to walk vigorously." This makes sense, because I've had some hikes that turned into yikes when spotting a snake on the trail or running into a cobweb.

Jump forward to 1809 and we have the first recorded uses of "hyke" with a Y as an English dialect word, also meaning "to walk vigorously." Unlike the act of hiking itself, "hyke" with a Y didn't go very far and didn't gain widespread status until the early 1900s. That's when it got a modern makeover to "hike" with an I and people started using it to describe long walks in the countryside.

Dictionaries offer a couple definitions for hike: (1) a long walk especially for pleasure or exercise; (2) an upward movement; rise

While I like the first definition, I love the second one. Because it also describes the inspirational feeling you get from hiking. That upward movement in your spirit. The elation of gaining elevation and getting that panoramic view from the top. Just like Francesco Petrarca did.

## **WALKING AROUND THE WORLD**

Of course not everyone everywhere uses the word "hiking." Depending on where in the world your feet are moving, you might be calling it something completely different.

A little research points out how far those words can wander.

"Hiking" is commonly used to describe a long, energetic walk in the woods — if that walk is in North America and continental Europe.

Some countries — I'm looking at you UK and Ireland — simply call it "walking," whether it's an after-dinner stroll or an epic climb through the MacGillycuddy Reeks of Kerry. However, if you're an old-school hiker in the UK you might say you're "rambling" your way through the outdoors. I'm guessing the Allman Brothers would approve of that one.

"Trekking" is the word of choice if you're journeying through India, South America and parts of Africa. Or on the Starship Enterprise.

In Australia, you might be "bushwalking" while you explore the trail. However if you're a short 1500 kilometers from Australia, in New Zealand, you are "tramping." And I suppose if you are listening to my favorite 70s band while doing it, you are... "Supertramping."

The point is, there are many ways to describe this wonderful wander. And all the world loves it.

## Millions of Miles to Explore

Our friends at AllTrails list an astonishing 400,000+ trails worldwide. In over 150 countries. That's a lotta miles...or kilometers, depending on where your boots are at the time.

I've had the pleasure of hiking some of the top trails out there (more on my favorite hikes in Chapter 6), but I've only scratched the surface. The bucket list for my boots just keeps growing.

## WELLNESS IN THE WOODS

I'd love to visit the Overland Track in Australia, a challenging scramble through Tasmania's untamed wilderness. The Kumano Kodo in Japan, (a UNESCO World Heritage Site) that winds its way through mountains and forests, with stops at ancient shrines and temples. The Tour du Mont Blanc, surrounding the Alps' highest peak, which takes you through France, Italy and Switzerland. Canada's West Coast Trail, with breathtaking ocean views off Vancouver Island. And the comically named Trolltunga ("Troll Tongue") in Norway, with scenic trails that lead you to a thin rock formation jutting out from the cliff like a troll's tongue, 3600 feet above sea level.

Here in the U.S., our passion for climbing trails continues to climb. According to a 2023 Outdoor Participation Trends Report from the Outdoor Industry Association, hiking is the most popular outdoor activity across America. The group estimates there are now nearly 60 million hikers in the U.S. Fortunately, they're not all on the same trail you are at the same time.

I live across from Washington Park in Portland. Washington Park is connected to Forest Park which has a huge network of trails. I try to get there four to five days a week. My

## DAVID HENTHORNE

favorite trail is the Wildwood Trail. **– John, Oregon**

North Cheyenne Cañon Park is a city park just ten minutes from my house in Colorado Springs. This canyon winds alongside a serene creek and offers dozens of trails that range from moderate to difficult. I like hiking here in the morning before the crowds hit. My favorite is a five mile round trip trek from the nature center up to the summit of Mount Custer, which overlooks Colorado Springs to the east and the foothills of the Rockies to the west.
**– Hannah, Colorado**

America has tens of thousands of awesome trails, each with its own challenges and rewards. While most of the top hikes are in our national parks (thank you, Teddy Roosevelt), don't overlook the wonderful wanders waiting in state parks, city parks, nature preserves and even private lands.

Some of the most popular U.S. trails year after year include the usual suspects:
- Angels Landing Trail and The Narrows, Zion National Park, Utah

- Devil's Bridge Trail via Dry Creek Road, Coconino National Forest, Arizona
- Half Dome, Yosemite National Park, California
- Navajo Loop and Queens Garden Trail, Bryce Canyon National Park, Utah
- Vernal and Nevada Falls via Mist Trail, Yosemite National Park, California
- Skyline Trail, Mount Rainier National Park, Washington
- Delicate Arch, Arches National Park, Utah
- Emerald Lake Trail, Rocky Mountain National Park, Colorado
- Highline Trail, Glacier National Park, Montana
- Acadia Mountain in Acadia National Park, Maine
- Bright Angel Trail in Grand Canyon National Park, Arizona
- Mount Whitney in Sequoia National Park, California

So, with all these epic trails, where in the world do you get started?

DAVID HENTHORNE

    The where doesn't matter nearly as much as the when. The sooner the better.

# "THE MOUNTAINS ARE CALLING AND I MUST GO."

— JOHN MUIR

## Chapter 2

# If we want more Father Time on our side, we need more Mother Nature

*A walk in the woods does a body good. Science says so.*

First things first, a disclaimer: I'm not a doctor. I can't give medical advice. But I can share the research I've done and how hiking has helped me. And it has. Helped me body, mind and soul. But please don't use this book as a replacement for real advice from a trusted medical professional. Web-MD does not count. It's always a good idea to consult a real doctor before beginning any new exercise program. There, I said it.

Hiking makes you feel good. That's not just me saying it, that's science. And who are we to contradict science? I'm sure Bill Nye the Science Guy would have a lot to say about the scientific evidence of healthy hiking.

*Fun fact:* Bill Nye the Science Guy once took me for a ride in his electric car. I was at a pitch meeting in Los Angeles about potentially using him in a big advertising campaign. After the meeting he insisted on taking me for a spin in his brand new EV. This was long before Electric Vehicles were a common thing. Before Tesla was a billion dollar glimmer in Elon's eye. Bill was the first person I met who owned one, or even considered owning one. And he sure was proud of it. I'll never forget the mischievous look in Bill Nye's eyes as he warned, "Hold on!" He punched the accelerator with grinning glee and laughed maniacally as we immediately — and quietly — flew down Hollywood Boulevard.

As Bill Nye and his science crew would no doubt agree, there is strong empirical data about the health and wellness benefits of hiking in the woods. It's a great way to get moving and improve your physical health. It's a weight-bearing exercise, so it helps strengthen your bones and muscles. Hiking can help improve your cardiovascular health, balance, and coordination. And because it is a low-impact activity, it can be enjoyed by kids, seniors, and everyone in between. Four-legged family members too.

# "Walking is man's best medicine."

— Hippocrates

## Sitting is quitting

I found a staggering stat when researching for this book. According to a 2022 study from the Center for Disease Control, about 25% of American adults are considered "physically inactive." And over 60% of U.S. adults don't engage in the recommended amount of activity. Of course there are plenty of adults with health and mobility issues who simply aren't able to move, or move enough. But for most of us, we're just too damn sedentary for our own good. We screen and we scroll and we make a permanent indentation on the sofa. All that physical inactivity leads to serious health problems including heart disease, diabetes, cancer, obesity and more. And the older we get, the worse it gets.

But we don't have to sit there and take it. We can do something about it. For me, and hopefully you if you're reading this, that something is hiking.

While you probably don't need a scientific study to convince you that hiking is good for your health, there are a gigaton of them out there. One published in the journal *Heart* found that hiking was associated with a lower risk of death from all causes, including heart disease. A study from *Diabetes Care* showed that hiking was associated with a lower risk of developing type 2 diabetes, a chronic disease that affects how your body metabolizes sugar. Another study, published in the journal *Gait & Posture*, found that hiking was associated with improved balance and gait in older adults. Balance and gait problems are common in older adults and can increase the risk of falls. And a study in the *Journal of the American Heart Association* provides strong evidence that hiking can improve circulation. Want your blood to keep moving? Then get moving.

## How hiking improves your physical health

**Hiking improves cardiovascular health.** Hiking is a great way to strengthen your heart muscle, improve your circulation, and lower your blood pressure and cholesterol. That's all good stuff. Because better cardio fitness helps your heart, lungs and blood vessels work together as a cohesive team to deliver oxygen to your muscles. Go Team, Go! All that teamwork helps reduce your risk of heart attack, stroke and other cardiovascular diseases. In other words, your heart will <3 you.

A 2021 scientific study published in the *Journal of Strength and Conditioning Research* concluded that hiking can increase your peak oxygen uptake, which is an important part of your overall cardiovascular fitness. Which means better endurance and a reduced risk of cardiovascular diseases like heart attack and stroke.

**Hiking builds stronger bones and muscles.** Hiking is a weight-bearing activity, which means it's building your body in important ways. It engages different muscle groups, helping to build strength and endurance. A 2018 study in the *International Journal of Sports Medicine* found that when we hike regularly, we're improving the strength in our lower body, including our calves, quads and hamstrings. And while you might not get ripped or shredded or swole, you're building strong muscles and bones for the long walk of life.

How does hiking pump you up? Hiking causes your muscles to work against gravity, which helps to build muscle mass. Muscle mass is important for bone health because it helps to support and protect those bones. Hiking also increases the amount of stress on your bones, which triggers the body to build new bone tissue. This helps to increase bone density and reduce the risk of osteoporosis. And because you're often walking on uneven terrain, hiking helps improve your balance and coordination. This is important for preventing falls (especially as you get older) which can lead to bone fractures.

Want to up your muscle and bone building potential? Carry a backpack. It adds weight to your hike, which can help strengthen muscles and bones. Plus, you'll be glad you brought the sunscreen, bug spray, headlamp and healthy snacks inside. Start with a light backpack and gradually increase the weight as you get stronger.

Hiking improves my cardio health, strengthens my legs and core, and increases blood flow. If I have sore muscles, one of the best things I can do to feel better is take a moderate hike. **– Lisa, Ohio**

## WELLNESS IN THE WOODS

Hiking, especially at 6500 ft and above where I live, has done wonders for my endurance and cardiovascular strength. I wear zero-drop shoes when I hike, which strengthen the small muscles of the foot, the ankles, and the calves. **– Hannah, Colorado**

It keeps me active and is part of a routine for me. Living so close to the park I don't really have an excuse not to hike. I end up having streaks going and it becomes a bit of a competition internally to push myself. As a result I feel better physically. Plus it's the time in nature, experiencing peace and solitude. Having the opportunity to exercise in beautiful surroundings. **– John, Oregon**

**Hiking helps weight loss.** We've all seen the incredible promises of a thinner tomorrow. Your Instagram and Facebook feed are chock full of them. "Sleep the pounds away! Get shredded overnight! Lose that belly fat for good!" There are a million weight-loss fads and fasts and schemes and scams but in the end, it just comes down to putting in the work. Exercise regularly, eat a healthy diet. Calories burned > calories consumed.

Hiking can help you burn those calories and lose weight. It's a low-impact approach that ignites your calorie-burn and builds muscle. The number of calories burned while hiking depends on a number of factors, such as your weight, the distance you hike, the intensity, and the elevation gain. However, most people burn between 200 and 400 calories per hour. Here's a bonus boost: It can also help reduce stress and improve your mood, which can make it a heck of a lot easier to stick to that healthy diet and exercise plan.

Our science friends are back again recommending the trail. A 2019 study in the *Journal of the American Medical Association* concluded that adults who participated in nature-based activities, like hiking, burned more calories than folks who exercised indoors. Another study, from the journal *Medicine & Science in Sports & Exercise*, found that hiking was more effective than walking for burning calories. And a study published in the journal *Applied Physiology, Nutrition, and Metabolism* found that hiking helped reduce body fat percentage and waist circumference.

Personally, I've found that I burn more calories hiking than reading scientific studies.

**Hiking improves balance and coordination.** Balance and coordination are essential skills for everyday life. They help us to walk, climb stairs, play sports, dance the limbo and other essential activities. As we age, our balance and coordination can naturally decline. Hiking is a great way to help maintain them, because it requires you to navigate uneven terrain, avoid obstacles -- and not fall off cliffs.

A study published in the journal *Physical Therapy in Sport* found that hiking was more effective than other types of exercise, such as walking and strength training, for improving balance and coordination in older adults. Another study, from the *Journal of Aging and Physical Activity*, found that hiking helped to improve balance and coordination in people with Parkinson's disease.

According to our scientist friends, hiking also helps improve your proprioception, the sense of where your body is in space, by forcing you to pay attention to your body position and movement. Another thing that forces you to pay attention is trying to pronounce "proprioception."

**Hiking reduces fatigue.** Let's face it, we're all exhausted. All the time. Too many tasks, not enough hours in the day. We're wiped out. But the juice we need isn't always in a can of Redbull or a shot of espresso. It's in the hills and on the trails.

Hiking can help reduce fatigue and improve your energy levels, because it gets your heart rate up, increases your oxygen intake and improves your circulation. It can also help reduce stress because exercise releases those precious endorphins and their mood-boosting effects.

A study published in the journal *Medicine & Science in Sports & Exercise* found that hiking was more effective than other types of exercise, such as walking and strength training, for reducing fatigue in people with chronic fatigue syndrome. A study from *Environmental Science & Technology* reports that hiking in a forest was associated with a reduction in fatigue levels in healthy adults.

Now some of you might be thinking, "How can hiking reduce my fatigue if I'm too fatigued to start hiking?" Not surprisingly, it's like any exercise advice: Start slow. Choose a shorter trail and gradually increase the distance and difficulty as you get stronger. It's ok to take your time, just take that first step.

**Hiking may even bolster immune systems.** While all the facts aren't in yet, recent research suggests that hiking may also have potential immune system benefits. A 2020 study in the journal *Frontiers in Immunology* found that regular exposure to nature, and exercise in it, can increase the activity of natural "killer cells," which are key in our immune defenses. So hiking might be even healthier than we think.

**Hiking improves joint health and flexibility.** Joint pain seems inescapable for most people. Fortunately, hiking is here to help. It's a low-impact activity that's easy on your joints, and also helps strengthen the muscles around them for added support. It lubricates your joints, reducing friction and pain, and reduces inflammation. And it improves your range of motion, making your joints more flexible and less painful.

The scientific studies have a lot to say about this one. A 2018 study in the journal *Arthritis Care & Research* concluded that low-impact hiking helped improve knee joint health and reduce pain in individuals with osteoarthritis. A study published in the journal *Osteoarthritis and Cartilage* found that hiking was associated with a reduced risk of developing osteoarthritis. The smart folks at *Rheumatology International* found that hiking was effective for improving joint range of motion and reducing pain.

But none of those studies can tell me more than my own knees have.

## THE DAY MY JOINTS JUMPED FOR JOY

A few years ago when knee pain made trail running a true challenge, I shifted from running through the woods to hiking through them. I still admire those who can set out on a good trail run, whether 5k sprinters or experienced ultra-marathoners. My daughter Hannah has completed several marathons, triathlons and 50k trail runs. A 50k is a whopping 31 miles of roots and rocks. One time, she even did it after spraining her ankle five miles in. Meaning she sprained her ankle – and then ran a marathon. Impressive doesn't begin to describe it.

But for me, it was time to give my knees a break. Bad knees and loss of cartilage run in my family (thanks, Dad) and it was my time. I wasn't ready to get knee surgery just yet, but I was ready to modify my exercise routine.

Hiking's low impact and slower pace made a huge difference to my joint pain. But more than that, taking my time gave me something even deeper. I saw the woods — and felt them — in a whole new way. Saw light dappling through the leaves in a way I never had. I heard the gentle sounds of the forest, and the relieved sighs of my knees.

## Scientific Journals, Personal Journeys

So there it is. Hiking helps your physical health. All those scientific journals say so.

But unlike more extreme exercises that may not be appropriate for your fitness level, hiking lets you do it at your own pace. Even light hiking can raise your heart rate to a moderate level, which helps to strengthen your heart and lungs. If you ask me (and Google) how to get the most health benefits from hiking, it's best to do it regularly and at a moderate intensity. What's that mean? A moderately intense workout will make you breathe a bit harder and work up a light sweat, but still allow you to still talk without gasping. That's the sweet spot. Plus, you're more likely to stick with a program that you don't come to dread.

## WELLNESS IN THE WOODS

How can you get the most health benefits from your hike?

- Try to hit the trail at least 3x per week, for at least 30 minutes each time. While my ideal hike is 3-13 miles, just getting out there for a quick half hour on a regular basis has big benefits.

- Warm up before you start hiking by walking slowly for a few minutes. Pick up the pace when you're ready, or depending on the challenge of the terrain.

- Cool down after you've "crossed the finish line." Walk slowly for a few minutes and don't forget to stretch. You can't underestimate the importance of stretching, after any exercise really. Especially the older you get and depending on the distance you've trekked. Those muscles just got you there and back, show them a little love.

- Hydrate like your future depends on it. Because it does. Drink plenty of water before, during, and after your hike.

- It is also important to choose a hiking trail that is appropriate for your fitness level. If you are new to hiking, start with a shorter trail and gradually increase the distance and difficulty of the trails you hike as you get stronger.

- Lastly, listen to your body. If you are feeling pain or pushing yourself beyond your comfort level, stop and rest. Don't be afraid to take breaks. It's better to take a break than to push yourself too hard and risk getting injured. Give yourself permission to go slowly and win at your own pace.

## *Hike Hack: Cross-training on the trail*

Hiking is great exercise for cardio, calorie burn, increased heart health, building balance and core strength, and a million other reasons. But sometimes you crave even a little more work in your workout. On those times I like to add in some cross-training for variety and overall fitness.

Many walking and hiking trails have exercise stations or obstacles along the path. They're called various things — fitness trails, workout trails, parcourses –– but whatever name they're called, they all feature exercise stops at regular intervals. These stations offer different physical challenges: sit-ups, pull-ups, balance beam, rope ladders, tire flips, and whatever else the trail designer can imagine. It's a fun way to break up the miles and tax your muscles in a different way.

But what if you're hiking a trail without any exercise stations, and still want that multi-muscle burn? No sweat. Just takes a little creativity.

## WELLNESS IN THE WOODS

Here's one of my favorite cross-training tricks, at one of my favorite parks.

I love hiking at Highbanks MetroPark on the northside of Columbus. It's a perennial favorite for nature lovers in central Ohio, winning annual readers' polls as "favorite local park." It's also a mere mile from my ad agency office. I've logged more miles there than any other park I suppose. Whether it's a pre-work wander, lunch-time trail run, or after-work workout.

Highbanks gets its name from its most unique feature, the steep banks overlooking the Olentangy River. Over 100 feet tall. It's quite a view from up there, especially since bald eagles started nesting along the river below a few years ago. Highbanks has ten challenging trails, an awesome nature center, and several ancient earthworks and burial mounds from the indigenous Adena culture.

What it didn't have was exercise stations. At least not official ones. But it does have benches throughout the trails. There are some high hills heading to those high banks and people often stop to catch their breath after a climb.

When I'm hiking there and want that extra push, I stop at every bench and turn it into an improv exercise station. Usually 25 pushups at each bench. Or sometimes alternating between pushups and tricep dips. Depending on which trail you take, those benches (and exercises) can really add up, totaling 300-500 or more. It's exhausting but worth it, even if you get some funny looks from folks out for a nature stroll.

DAVID HENTHORNE

## *Hike Hack: Burn calories without burning out*

You definitely blaze through some calories when you're blazing a trail. Depending on the duration and intensity of your hike, those calories can add up quickly. And that's a good thing. Here are a few tips for tipping the scales in your favor.

There are plenty of fitness apps that can help you track the total calorie burn. My favorite is "Map-MyRun," which is owned by UnderArmor. Even though it's called MapMyRun you can select from a variety of exercises on a drop-down menu. I use it when I hike, bike, trail run, even on an elliptical or stationary bike. I can't guarantee the 100% accuracy of the app's calorie count, but it's a big-time reward to see those big numbers at the end of a long hike. And a great motivator for the next one. Watching that calorie count also encourages you to go the extra mile –– or few hundred feet even –– to hit a higher number before ending the hike. No one wants to stop at 1299 calories when you could hit 1300. It's the equivalent of "one more rep" at the gym.

For extra calorie burn I like to wear a backpack with some weight in it. Not an 80-pound pack for ascending Everest, but even a few extra pounds of gear and essentials will add to the challenge. Besides, you'll want to pack that backpack with a healthy lunch and snacks to eat during the hike. Go for fruits, nuts, healthy trail bars, and quick protein. Peanut butter is a fan favorite, beef jerky too. Try to avoid processed or sugary foods. While you're burning calories it's important to refuel and add a few good ones back into your system, so you can avoid lightheadedness, dizziness and dehydration. Speaking of which, always bring plenty of water to keep your body functioning properly. Water helps you feel full and plays a role in weight loss.

# "IF I HAD KNOWN I WAS GOING TO LIVE THIS LONG, I'D HAVE TAKEN BETTER CARE OF MYSELF."

— Mickey Mantle

## Chapter 3

# Crooked trails help you think straight

*Why your brain wants you to take a hike*

Hiking is a great boost for our bodies, and our brains. Yes, in addition to plenty of physical benefits, a walk in the woods has a slew of mental health benefits too. Maybe, just maybe, that's why the human brain, with all its twisting ridges and grooves, looks more than a little like a winding trail map. Think about it the next time you see one.

### How hiking improves your mental health

**Hiking reduces stress and anxiety.** Spending time hiking in nature has been shown to reduce stress and anxiety levels. A 2018 study in the journal *Environmental Science & Technology* found that participants who spent time in nature reported lower levels of anxiety and depression. Another study in that same journal discovered that people who walked in a forest for 90 minutes had lower levels of the stress hormone cortisol than people who walked in an urban setting. And we should all say yes to less stress.

**Hiking improves mood.** Want to improve your mood, boost your self-esteem and reduce feelings of depression? Hit the trail, because hiking releases endorphins and their mood-boosting effects. A study in the journal *Proceedings of the National Academy of Sciences* found that people who walked for 90 minutes in a natural area had increased activity in the brain region associated with positive emotions. But wait there's more. Hiking can also help you connect with nature, appreciate the beauty of your surroundings, and spark your curiosity to learn more about the world around you.

**Hiking improves cognitive function and memory.** Not only does hiking offer a chance to make great memories in nature, it can actually help our memory itself. A 2016 study in the journal *Environmental Science & Technology* concluded that spending time in nature helped improve cognitive function and memory in older adults. Another study, in *Psychological Science*, found that people who hiked in the woods for 90 minutes had improved cognitive function on tests of memory, attention, and problem-solving skills. Hiking fires up your brain, requiring you to focus on your surroundings and navigate the uneven terrain. All that fresh air helps too.

Hiking is my best tool for stress management. I have a practice of not bringing my problems into the woods with me. I leave them at the trailhead and tell myself I can pick them back up on the way out, but I never want to. **– Carie, Ohio**

I feel very relaxed mentally even if I'm working hard on a difficult trail. It gets you away from all the electronics and life's daily pressures. **– Scott, Colorado**

I'm appreciative & thankful for the time I spend hiking. When I hike alone it's primarily a meditative experience for me. This allows me to clear my head and has great mental health benefits. When I hike with someone it usually results in a strong, meaningful conversation. **– John, Oregon**

Hiking allows me to take a break from the screens and clears my mind of clutter. Some of my most creative ideas have come to me while hiking! **– Lisa, Ohio**

Stepping outside of the everyday and into the natural world encourages creativity, contemplation, and curiosity. I wrap up a hike feeling grateful for the opportunity to exist alongside the natural world. **– Hannah, Colorado**

**Hiking improves sleep quality.** A good walk in the woods, especially at a longer distance, tires you out. And that's not a bad thing. The physical exertion and time in nature and natural light can result in better sleep. A 2019 study in the journal *Sleep Medicine* concluded that people who spent time in nature before bed drifted off faster and got deeper sleep, resulting in reduced stress and increased relaxation.

**Hiking boosts creativity and imagination.** Wandering the woods has long been recognized as a vital part of the creative process. It's been said that Ludwig van Beethoven went for a five hour walk every afternoon in the woods near Vienna, Austria. Friedrich Nietsche walked up to eight hours a day and even wrote, "All truly great thoughts are conceived by walking." Charles Darwin, Ernest Hemingway, Aristotle, Tchaikovsky, Thoreau (quoted at the beginning of this chapter) and so many other great thinkers knew that getting up and getting outside gets their creativity going.

Science knows it too. A study from Stanford University with the incredibly lengthy but absolutely perfect title, *"Give your Ideas some Legs: The Positive Effect of Walking on Creative Thinking,"* showed that walking boosts creativity during the activity itself, by 60% on average, and that boost continues for some time after. A study from the University of Utah found that backpackers scored 50% better on a creativity test when they were in nature vs. before the trip started. And according to research from the University of Illinois, brain activity for students taking a test after a 20-minute walk was much higher than for students who sat while the others walked. The lesson? If you just sit there, your brain will too.

So, can hiking actually make you smarter? With this much scientific evidence we'd be dumb not to find out.

## Finding the hiker's high

Everybody's heard the term "Runners' High," right? That deeply relaxing euphoria you feel after a long run or lengthy aerobic exercise. People who experience a runner's high also feel less anxiety and pain right afterwards. Is it the burst of endorphins released in the bloodstream, as researchers have long believed? Or, as new research suggests, could it be due to endocannabinoids, neurotransmitters in the brain that create feelings similar to cannabis (guess that's the hits-just-right "high" in a Runner's High).

Whatever scientists are pointing their euphoric finger at, something is telling your nervous system, "Man, this feels amazing." Runners often feel that beautiful bliss from sweaty head to tired toe.

I've found you can get that same elation sensation with a good hike. I'm a true believer in the "Hiker's High." For me, it usually hits around mile six or so. You're a couple hours in, feeling the effects. If it's an out-and-back, you've flip-turned like Michael Phelps for the last leg of the gold-medal journey. If it's a loop, you're on the "back nine," working your way back to the clubhouse. Either way, that Hiker's High hits your heart and head and lungs and legs and propels you the rest of the way, no matter the challenge. The checkered flag is within reach. Just make sure you stretch when you get to the end of the trail, especially if you've got a long drive back home. Otherwise, you'll stiffen up and walk like Fred Sanford from the car to your next stop.

## WHEN YOU WANDER YOUR MIND DOES TOO

As an advertising creative director, my entire career has been about developing creative ideas for commercials and campaigns. Whether it's a headline or a logo or a layout or a jingle, it starts with that little lightbulb popping on in your head.

Many of those creative ideas have popped into my mind while I'm traipsing the trail. Which is why I always pack a pen and notebook in addition to my iPhone so the idea doesn't hike right out of my head.

There's something about the elixir of fresh air, whispering winds, and pumping blood that sets your mind free. Gets the creative juices flowing. For me, the best ideas don't come when I'm facing a screen. They come surrounded by trees.

## Hike Hack: Stream...of consciousness

Bruce Lee famously said to move like water. The martial arts legend advised, "Empty your mind. Be formless. Shapeless. Like water. Water can flow, or it can crash. Be water, my friend."

One of my favorite Hike Hacks is stopping for a Mindfulness Moment at a rushing stream or babbling brook. Water sounds are naturally soothing, and the gurgle of running water has long been used in meditation practices. Apparently our brains are wired to perceive sounds as either threatening or nonthreatening –– and a gentle waterfall is the latter. Scientists say the smooth, steady sounds of moving water can guide our brain's neural waves to a calmer place, help reduce anxiety and heart rate, and even stimulate our parasympathetic nervous system. I just know it gives me a chill vibe.

## WELLNESS IN THE WOODS

I like to stand still...eyes closed...and just listen. As the water flows, so should your thoughts. Your creativity. Your imagination. Let your brain babble just like that brook. Try to silence the inner critic that judges thoughts too soon. Just let them flow. Water finds a way through that forest, just like it will through your mind.

# "I TOOK A WALK IN THE WOODS AND CAME OUT TALLER THAN THE TREES."

— HENRY DAVID THOREAU

DAVID HENTHORNE

## Chapter 4

# Let nature nurture your hurting heart

*How to find that healing feeling*

I played a lot of little league baseball as a kid. I wasn't great, but I wasn't half bad. Later in life when he was talking to my coworker friends, my father bluntly described my baseball skillset as "decent glove, no stick." Gee, thanks, Dad. While I don't think that's an entirely accurate assessment of my talents, those co-workers never let me live it down. But despite that underwhelming description, I was a good teammate, loved the sport, and would do anything to try to help us win.

For instance, one game when our regular (and only) catcher didn't show up, Coach asked which one of us wanted to step up to the plate. Or in this case, behind it.

## DAVID HENTHORNE

Looking up and down the dugout not one hand went up. No one wanted the job. With a healthy dose of disappointment Coach told us, "Look, if no one volunteers we have to forfeit the game." Still no one was willing to suit up. I'd never caught before but I could feel the clock ticking and wasn't about to let the game end without even starting. So of course I threw my hand up, put on the catcher's mask and gear, and crouched down behind the plate. Play ball!

A few innings went by and to my surprise it wasn't so bad. I was actually catching on to catching. It all started making sense. Until...it all went horribly wrong. This was little league player-pitch baseball, and after a few innings the pre-teen pitcher started running out of steam. The throws became erratic. Wide of home plate, or brushing back the batter. And worst of all...short pitches hitting in front of the plate then taking wild hops. One of those wild hops did exactly what a young man doesn't want it to do as he squats oh-so-vulnerably just inches above the ground.

Anyone who tells you an athletic cup will offer plenty of protection from a wild pitch in the dirt has never been on the receiving end of said pitch.

As I lay there writhing on my back in the dusty infield I looked over at my teammates and realized why no one else had raised their hand. I rubbed my knee in a vain attempt to trick the crowd into thinking the ball had hit me somewhere other than where it had. But based on the gasps and groans of the parents (especially the dads) they knew exactly where that brutal bounce had landed. It was more than just the physical hurt from that bad hop — it was also the embarrassment of it all. Somewhere through the haze and humiliation I heard my coach's gruff voice and old-school medical advice: "Walk it off."

I'd heard that phrase before. I'd certainly hear it plenty more times in the years to come. Just get up, get going, and walk it off. So I did. After a few agonizing minutes, and several cup adjustments, I was back in the game.

"Walk it off" was good guidance on the diamond that day. It's still good advice, because no matter what life throws at you, healing — both physical and emotional — can happen when you walk it off.

Spending time in nature helps you reset, flip the script, and reclaim your emotional tranquility. Stressful triggers are left behind with every step forward. This is hiking's superpower.

Got a worried mind or heavy heart? Walk it off.

## **NATURE HEALS ITSELF. IT CAN HEAL YOU TOO.**

Despite all kinds of obstacles, nature is pretty darn good at healing itself. We see it every year in the rebirth from winter's hibernation. We also see it when society pollutes and ravages a habitat. Thankfully, given time, as long as there are seeds and roots and soil and sun, an ecosystem can restore itself. We can be restored too.

Perhaps Dr. Ian Malcolm said it best. My favorite character in *Jurassic Park*, played by the black-clad and ever-cool Jeff Goldblum, sums it up perfectly with his take on the dinosaur disaster: "Life, finds a way."

While I've never encountered a T-Rex on the trail, I've overcome a demon or two. Frustrations, temptations, hurts and heartbreaks. I've left them all in the dust, miles behind me. There's never betrayal on the trail.

As nature embraces you and fresh air fills your lungs, you can feel the worry leave your body and a kind, calming effect takes over. I find that the more I wander outdoors, the more I find my inner peace.

When struggles creep in, that's the time to head out. Whether it's finances or family, health or heartbreak, hiking heals.

## THE SCIENCE AND THE SOUL

In addition to its substantial benefits on your physical and mental health, a walk in the woods can do wonders for your soul. It gives you the time and space to reflect, reframe and relax. Hiking helps reduce the production of cortisol, the stress hormone, easing those gnawing feelings of anxiety. It also releases that extremely dope dopamine we all crave, improving your mood, boosting self-esteem, and reducing depression. Importantly, wandering the woods can also enhance our ability to find meaning and purpose in life. Time in nature connects us to something larger than ourselves, and fosters a greater sense of well-being.

**Hiking reduces rumination and negative self-focus.** No doubt we all go down the rabbit hole of rumination. That spiral of negative thinking and worry. Our brains seem to love dwelling on what's bad, what's wrong, what's never going to happen. In a 2015 study published in the *Proceedings of the National Academy of Sciences* (one of the world's most prestigious research journals), Stanford researchers concluded that a 90-minute walk in the woods, compared to an urban walk, significantly reduced dwelling on these negative thoughts. With its healthy challenges and exposure to nature, hiking helps reduce harmful rumination and tells those negative thoughts to, you guessed it, take a hike.

**Hiking improves our positive emotions.** Not surprisingly, a healthy hike not only reduces our bad feelings, it also increases our good ones. Once again, the balance of nature. A study published in the *Journal of Environmental Psychology* showed that spending time trekking the trails boosts our positive emotions and overall well-being. Making our feelings...*feel* better. In other words, hiking can make us happy.

**Hiking increases our mindfulness.** Focusing on the sights, sounds and sensations during our woods walks and reducing distractions (i.e. Put your phone away) can boost our mindfulness and overall well being. A 2018 study in *Frontiers in Psychology* found that time in nature can help boost our present-moment awareness and reduce stress. Plus, when you're climbing that precarious cliff and your legs and lungs are burning, you gotta be in the moment.

**Hiking improves self-esteem and resilience.** According to a 2019 study in the *Journal of Environmental Psychology*, researchers found that participants who finished a challenging hike reported increased self-esteem and an overall sense of accomplishment. It's true, conquering challenges on the trail builds resilience and confidence in life.

**Hiking builds social connections and reduces loneliness.** For many, hiking is a terrific solo pursuit, but there are also proven benefits of hiking with others. A 2018 study in the *International Journal of Environmental Research and Public Health* found that participating in group hikes has a major impact on creating social connections and reducing feelings of loneliness. Hey, in these times of increased isolation (pandemic hangover, remote work, online addictions), getting outside for a good old-fashioned group hike can be a valuable way to knock the lonely off and improve your sense of belonging.

# WELLNESS IN THE WOODS

Hiking is a major stress reducer. Hiking humbles me. It reminds me that no matter how big a problem I am facing, the world, and my life, will go on. **– Lisa, Ohio**

I've turned to hiking to help my mental state. It has helped me through the end of a marriage, and the loss of two siblings and a very close friend. **– John, Oregon**

It's hard to describe the healing power of the woods, but it's there for those who are looking for it. **– Carie, Ohio**

When I was recovering from chemo, my daily hikes helped me feel like I was working toward regaining my life before cancer. As the years went by and my strength improved, mentally I moved to being a cancer survivor versus a cancer patient. **– Scott, Colorado**

DAVID HENTHORNE

## Harmony inside and out: the yoga/hiking connection

In this fast-paced world, the journey to wellness takes many paths. Interestingly, two seemingly far apart activities — hiking and yoga — share surprising similarities and a powerful combination of benefits to help us find that well-being. Whether you're hoofing it on a nature trail or downward dogging on a yoga mat, you can find a sense of balance, strength and connection.

**Connecting breath to movement.** At the core of both yoga and hiking lies the important relationship between breath and movement. Every yoga instructor I've ever heard emphasizes the importance of mindful breathing during every pose. Well it's the same when you're on the trail. Hiking encourages a deeper, rhythmic breathing pattern as you navigate the terrain. This synchronized breathing calms the mind, lowers stress hormones, and optimizes oxygen intake, improving overall well-being.

**Building flexibility and strength.** Yoga postures target different muscle groups, promoting strength, flexibility, and balance. Guess what? Hiking does too. Climbing those inclines works the legs and core, while uneven terrain challenges your balance and coordination. Over time, both practices can lead to improved posture, increased stamina, and a reduction in aches and pains.

**A sanctuary for the mind.** The repetitive nature of both yoga and hiking can be meditative. In yoga, focusing on the breath and the physical sensations of each pose quiets the mind and reduces anxiety. Similarly, the rhythmic steps of a hike and the repetitive motions of walking lull the mind into a state of present-moment awareness. This allows worries to fade away, leaving you with a sense of calmness and clarity.

**Embracing nature's embrace.** Yoga often incorporates imagery and metaphors of the natural world. Even the names of poses evoke nature: mountain pose, tree pose, lizard, cobra, rabbit, fish and more. Hiking, of course, takes you directly into nature's embrace. Both practices allow you to disconnect from digital devices and reconnect with the natural world. The sights and sounds of nature — the rustling leaves, the chirping birds, the sun on your skin — have a profound effect on reducing stress and promoting feelings of peace and well-being.

**A journey of self-discovery.** Yoga poses can challenge your body and reveal areas that require improvement. This fosters a sense of self-awareness and encourages you to reach your full potential. Hiking can also be a journey of self-discovery. As you navigate the trail, you push your physical and mental limits, fostering a sense of accomplishment and boosting confidence.

**A journey for all levels.** Yoga has a wide variety of styles, from gentle and restorative to vigorous and challenging. Anyone who thinks yoga can't be a tough workout hasn't done much yoga. Similarly, hiking trails can range from flat paved paths suitable for beginners to ridiculously strenuous climbs for the most experienced hikers. The key is to find a practice that suits your fitness level and allows you to experience the benefits at a level that's right for you.

**Putting the two together.** While the two activities can certainly be enjoyed separately, there are powerful benefits in combining your yoga mat and your hiking boots. That synergy creates a truly holistic approach to wellness. Yoga before your hike can improve flexibility, minimize injury risk, and center you for a more mindful experience. Post-hike yoga can help release tension, improve mobility, and aid your body in a quicker recovery.

## Brave Steps Toward a Better Life

I grew up visiting parks with my family. We visited, we picnicked, we camped. When they were younger, I took my own kids on so many mini-woods walks. I even had a teenage job working at a park snack shack. But I didn't start hiking seriously until after my mother died. I was in need of some deep healing, and hiking the deep woods offered that.

I thought about the life she had, the dreams she had, and how different her life would have been if her own mother hadn't taken some very brave steps.

Edith Bayless didn't leave Ashland, Kentucky...she escaped it.

What would push a young mother in Appalachian coal country to pack up her young daughter and flee 121 miles to the north? What situation drove her to uproot her life, leave her husband, and pray for a fresh start? It was never fully discussed in my family why my grandmother Edith left Kentucky, but the whispers said plenty.

She went looking for a better life. A safe life. For herself, and especially her young daughter Carolyn. Fortunately Edith found work as a live-in maid and nanny for a welcoming, well-to-do family in Columbus, the Madisons. Her daughter was even embraced and raised as a "sister" to the family's own daughter, Cindy. They grew up as best friends and remained that until my mother's passing in 2011.

Eventually Edith found love again. With a handsome and wholesome Ohio Highway Patrolman. Clarence Young was born and raised in Delaware, Ohio and was a proud veteran of World War II, where he served in the South Pacific theater. Later in life he shared stories and souvenirs with me from his time in the Fiji Islands. He talked of his time at

Guadalcanal. There's even the tale of him stationed on a South Pacific island and another sailor on that same island who went on to a great deal of fame. That navy man was John F. Kennedy.

When Clarence returned from the war, he put his navy communication skills to work with the Ohio Highway Patrol, where he served as a radio dispatcher for over 30 years. My Papaw was a larger than life character. Maybe my first hero. With his large frame, patrolman uniform and war stories he gave off serious John Wayne vibes. And while he wasn't a sports fan per se, he went by Cy instead of Clarence. Cy Young. My baseball buddies all did a double take when I introduced him that way.

Cy Young was indeed a hero. Because he provided for that young Kentucky mother and daughter and raised Carolyn like his own. Although never wealthy, they lived a rich life. Their home was filled with love and laughter. Mamaw Edith found a better life, 121 miles north and a world away.

Like most people of their time, my mother and grandmother had challenging lives filled with adversity. But they overcame them. They got up, moved forward, and healed the hurt. They never actually sat me down and gave me that advice. They didn't have to. I saw it in the way they lived life every day. When the climb got tough, they toughed it out. Their strength and courage and resolve keep me moving forward too.

## Hike Hack: Listen to your mother

Just like our own moms, Mother Nature usually has good advice. We just have to be willing to listen. The woods are full of wisdom, if we put our pride aside and pick up what they're putting down.

Next time on the trail, unplug your earbuds and get connected. Stop your hike and just listen to nature's lessons in benevolence and balance. What will you hear? The hard work and persistence of a hungry squirrel shooshing through the fallen leaves. The ingenuity of water winding its way to a peaceful place. The gentle creak of a tall tree who never stops striving. The cooperative communication of warbling songbirds. In this healing moment keep your mind — and your ears — tuned in to what this Mother is trying to tell you.

## *Hike Hack: Walking meditation*

Life comes at us fast. And we zoom through most of it, rushing and racing to fit everything in. But sometimes when we need healing the most, it's ok to just...be.

Next time you take a woods walk, take a mindful moment to simply feel the ground under your feet. Concentrate on your connection to the Earth. The trail under your boots. How it supports you, elevates you. Feel its strength and energy flowing up to you. Tune into your breath. Inhale and exhale slowly, deeply. Bring your focus to each step as you walk. How your heel feels when it hits the ground. How your body feels as you move through nature. Your striding legs, swinging arms, muscles and joints, all working as one. Listen for the sound your boots make when they touch the path.

Let nature in. Be totally present in the moment.

The woods can help us slow down and find the calm we need, in our time of need. Maybe stop moving for a moment and close your eyes. Listen to your body. Sit in the stillness if it's what your body is asking for. Close your eyes if it feels right. Disconnect from what troubles you. This mindful moment should be restful and restorative.

Once you've enjoyed this reset, for as long as you wish, continue on your journey. See your surroundings with fresh eyes and an open heart. Be receptive to the wonders around you, with a renewed sense of well-being.

# "And into the forest I go, to lose my mind and find my soul."

# WELLNESS IN THE WOODS

— John Muir

CHAPTER 5

# More caring boot prints, less carbon footprint

*An eco-friendly approach to hiking*

Anyone remember Ranger Rick? The friendly cartoon raccoon mascot of the National Wildlife Federation? As a kid I was all about Ranger Rick and couldn't wait to get the monthly magazine where he and his animal friends entertained and educated about the importance of nature. They cleaned up the pond and the park and the woods and all worked together as one big forest family. Back then I had no idea what a conservationist or environmentalist or eco-warrior was, but it sure made me care.

WELLNESS IN THE WOODS

I've tried to instill a bit of that Earth-friendly energy in my own kids. We mini-hiked a lot when they were younger, trying to fit in as many "woods walks" as we could after school and on weekends. We visited city parks and state parks and national parks. We appreciated every class of animal and type of tree. It must have sunk into their spongey little brains somehow, because they're now talking the talk and walking the (woods) walk as environmentally-conscious young adults.

After graduating with a botany degree, my son is a plant-loving professional horticulturist at Columbus' prestigious Franklin Park Conservatory, and a long-time vegan who just might save the world. My daughter is an outdoors-obsessed trail athlete, wandering the world by hike and bike and writing about her excellent adventures. They both value the wonders of nature and do more than their share to promote sustainability.

### THINKING GREEN AND HIKING CLEAN

In earlier chapters you heard about the scientifically-proven wellness benefits of hiking. While hitting the trails can do a lot for our health, it's also important to think about the health of the environment we're exploring. A good walk in the woods can connect you to the natural world — and inspire you to protect it.

For me, hiking has been the best way to appreciate the beauty of nature and the plants and animals that call it home. While we can learn a lot about nature by visiting museums and watching NatGeo videos, there's no better way to love it than by walking through it. Surrounded by the sights, sounds and smells of a living, breathing biome. That forest will give back to you, helping to reduce stress, improve your mood, and boost your well-being.

## How to be an Eco-Friendly Hiker:

**Leave no trace.** This is a big one. Actually a lot of big ones. There are plenty of leave no trace principles to follow that help minimize your impact on the environment. These range from disposing of waste properly to controlling campfires to using reusable water bottles and eco-friendly gear. Pack out what you pack in. In other words, leave it like you found it. Maybe even better than you found it. Pick up any trash on the trail and take it out with you. A debris-free trail is a happy trail.

**Stick to the trail.** Hiking trails are built and blazed for our own safety — and to protect the environment they run through and avoid habitat degradation. Where we step matters, so it's important to be mindful. When we go off trail we risk trampling on tender plants, or even tiny creatures. We wouldn't park our car on someone else's lawn. Plus, going off trail can potentially create a new path and plenty of confusion for future hikers...and AllTrails users.

WELLNESS IN THE WOODS

**Respect plants and wildlife.** We are just visiting these woods and trails, but others live here. Plants and animals can be greatly impacted by our actions. As tempting as it might be, don't pick that beautiful wildflower or interrupt that forest creature's foraging. Leave them to thrive in their natural habitat. And so that others may discover these natural wonders for themselves.

**Care enough to learn more.** Curious about what lives where you're hiking? Most parks and preserves have a nature center and on-site naturalists or volunteers to share the stories of that area's specific species. Take the time to ask them a question or three about what makes their region special. You won't be disappointed.

**Practice Kindness.** This goes for how you treat your fellow hikers (a friendly smile goes a long way to building forest fellowship) and how you treat nature itself. The woods deserve our kindest care.

> I feel energized when I hike. And full of gratitude for the beauty this world still holds for us despite all we've done to destroy it. **– Lisa, Ohio**

DAVID HENTHORNE

**IF WE HUG TREES, THEY'LL HUG US BACK**

I'm not sure how or when "tree hugger" became such a derogatory term. Some folks use it to derisively describe those they feel are obsessed, overly-protective environmentalists. But respecting and protecting the environment is the most important thing we can do. For our now and our next.

Fortunately, tree huggers seem to be standing taller than ever. In united groves of like-minded eco-warriors. You see the term more and more on social posts and t-shirts and badges and bumper stickers (often on a Prius). Those badges are a badge of honor, proudly proclaiming their owners' willingness to nurture nature. And we need nature to be healthy, for our own survival. If we take care of our forests and keep our woods well, they'll keep us well.

**ON A MISSION TO REGENERATE NATURE**

There are plenty of eco-friendly organizations doing important work for the greater good of the planet. Most are familiar names with large national or international networks. One such organization I've had the honor of working with is the California Academy of Sciences.

WELLNESS IN THE WOODS

Founded in 1853 and located in San Francisco's Golden Gate Park, the California Academy of Sciences (calacademy.org) is one of the world's leading research institutes and natural history museums. The architecturally stunning museum features an aquarium, planetarium, rainforest, and 46 million specimens, all under one living roof of indigenous plants.

It's an impressive place, with an equally impressive mission: "To regenerate the natural world through science, learning, and collaboration." To make nature wilder and healthier again. In other words, to save the planet.

I'm proud of the work we've done to promote this ambitious initiative. We've developed creative campaigns and marketing messages —in San Francisco and beyond — that motivate others to join the cause. Because it takes the world to regenerate the Earth.

## JOIN AN ECO-CAUSE YOU CARE ABOUT

It seems like every time I look at my email inbox or Instagram feed there's another plea or three to help the environment. And that's a good thing. A very good thing. Because we need as many people sending as many messages as possible until it sinks in: Earth needs our help.

So I'll gladly go through requests from nonprofits like The Nature Conservancy, World Wildlife Fund, Greenpeace, Environmental Defense Fund, and others. Plus messages from nature-focused businesses like Public Lands, REI (creators of the powerful #OptOutside campaign), Patagonia, Subaru, Jeep and plenty more.

I like knowing when an organization has a soul and a true mission to help the environment — especially those that are committed to helping restore nature. If that matters to you too, there are so many ways to help. Donating to Earth-friendly causes, voting for eco-minded candidates, volunteering at park or beach or waterway cleanup days, even picking up trash on the trail. As small as those gestures may seem, together they add up and truly make a difference.

While these large national and international organizations are doing essential work, there are also plenty of local groups focused on taking care of our own backyard. The old adage, "Think Globally, Act Locally" is truer than ever. That's the path I've taken.

While I enjoy traveling far and wide to hike, most of my trail time has been here in Ohio. Especially at the impressive state parks system. Ohio has 76 stunning state parks, from the shores of Lake Erie up north to the banks of the Ohio River in the south. The terrain ranges from the Appalachian foothills in the east to the prairies in the west.

I love hiking in my home state. My girlfriend and I have traveled to and trekked through nearly 60 of Ohio's 76 state parks. So when I discovered there was a recently-created nonprofit dedicated to supporting Ohio's state parks, I wanted to be part of it.

After a few rounds of interviews I was named a board trustee of the Ohio State Parks Foundation (OhioStateParksFoundation.org). Our mission is to enhance, preserve and protect Ohio's state parks, with a focus on making the parks accessible for all. The Foundation has held events and raised funds to help create pollinator gardens of native species, add ADA-compliant kayak launches, build Storybook Trails with kid-friendly narratives winding through the woods, and many other ways to inspire a love of nature.

Being part of a statewide nonprofit has increased my passion for the parks and all the trails in them. It's encouraged me to wander farther and explore more. I've also enjoyed working with like-minded outdoor enthusiasts who care about a common cause.

## Hike Hack: Take pictures with your eyes

A friend of mine rarely stops to take photos. Oddly enough, he's a cinematographer. Maybe because his profession is filming for movies and commercials he just doesn't feel like snapping pics in his personal life. Or at least not as often as other people. He'll jokingly say, "I took a picture with my eyes."

## DAVID HENTHORNE

Sometimes when we're hiking this is the perfect approach to a mindful moment. Not every tree or trail is Insta-worthy. But they're still worthy.

Nature has many gifts that deserve our observation, and our gratitude. On your next hike stop and appreciate what you see. Walk for a few moments in silence as you give thanks for the natural resources –– the trees, the grasses, the lakes, the rivers –– that support us, and so many other species. Notice the amazing details in the veins of a leaf, the petals of a flower, or the texture in a rock outcropping. Take a deep breath, and take in all you see.

## "ONE TOUCH OF NATURE MAKES THE WHOLE WORLD KIN."

— WILLIAM SHAKESPEARE

## Chapter 6

# Taking the first steps

*How to become a happy hiker*

Let's be honest, hiking isn't hard. You don't need years of specialized training or amazing athletic ability or a 36 on your ACT. You just need a healthy dose of want-to.

But as simple as it seems, if you're a hiking newbie there are still a few things you should keep in mind before you just get up and go. I've researched a lot and hiked a lot, and I've picked up some helpful tips along the way. Here are just a few things to know before you head for the trail.

**GET THE RIGHT GEAR**

This is so important it gets its own chapter. From Yaktrax to healthy snacks to the perfectly packed backpack, the right gear can make all the difference in your day. We'll dive into what to wear, what to bring, and the gear to get in Chapter 7.

## Find the right trail for your fitness level

Most inexperienced runners wouldn't just go out and run a marathon. Or even a 10k. Yet that's what some beginners do when it comes to hiking. Because it's a slower pace than running, they figure they can handle any trail out there. But elevation, distance, trail conditions, equipment and their own fitness can impact the experience. Even a moderate hike on an ideal day can be tiring, and lessen your enthusiasm for next time.

Where can you find the right trail? Research to the rescue! I'm a big fan of the AllTrails app. They put over 400,000 trails from around the world in the palm of your hand, with info, maps, distances, photos, and helpful tips from fellow hikers. Trails are listed as Easy, Moderate or Hard, so you can find one that's right for your fitness, but also your enjoyment. Tackling a trail with lush forests or mysterious caves or a killer view makes it all worthwhile.

There are endless other options for finding your perfect path, from helpful guidebooks to millions of websites. Seriously, *millions*. In fact, I just

## WELLNESS IN THE WOODS

Googled "hiking trails near me" and got a staggering 901,000,000 results in half a second.

Of course you can always ask your assistant..."Alexa, find a moderately challenging 6-mile hike near me."

### Consider how much time you have

This isn't nearly as depressing as it sounds. Not how much time you have left on this planet, but how much time you can devote to the hike. Do you have a couple hours or a full day? Choose a distance that makes sense for your schedule. The average adult walking pace is about 3 mph, but your time may vary based on trail conditions, elevation gain, your fitness and fatigue, weather, and many other factors. Remember to add in travel time to and from the trailhead. And build in some rest time during the hike itself, especially if it's one you haven't done before or more challenging than you're used to.

### Know the terrain

Sometimes you find the trail you want. And sometimes the trail just finds you. But it's usually a good idea to know where you're going and what kind of terrain you'll tackle. Are you heading to the mountains, where you'll encounter plenty of bouldering up and down steep inclines? Or are you headed to the desert where you're trekking through loose sand, blistering sun and arid conditions? Is your trail through a thick forest that could be overgrown with vegetation and fallen timber? Or are you doing your best yeti impression and wandering a winter wonderland of slippery snow and ice?

Each biome comes with unique challenges (and signature rewards) that impact what you wear and what you should pack.

> For me a perfect hike is 50-60 degrees, a new trail, unknown adventures...and great snacks! **– Carie, Ohio**

> I like a distance that makes you tired while providing enough visual stimulation to keep you distracted while hiking. **– Scott, Colorado**

> My favorite kind of hike is following a trail along a riverbed or creek with enough challenging terrain to make me sweat a little. A nice waterfall or a bridge crossing a river is a bonus! **– Lisa, Ohio**

> For me, the perfect hike has three things. Micro-adventuring: Finding something new and unexpected in an everyday event. Challenge: Getting a good workout physical-

ly and overcoming a turnaround spot or noticing a familiar climb go from difficult to doable. The Beauty: I always bring my camera to capture the adventure. **– Hannah, Colorado**

### KNOW THE TRAIL BEFORE YOU HIT THE TRAIL.

Some trails are harder than others. That's true because of distance, elevation changes, and obstacles. But it's also true because some are confusing and not well-marked. While many trails have frequent trail map guideposts, or color-coded blazes on the trees (signaling that you're on the red trail or blue trail for instance), not all of them do. Maybe the blazes have faded. Or your location marker on the guidepost map is worn off. Often the most confusing of all is when several trails intersect and criss-cross each other. If you're not diligently alert, you can wander quite a ways before you realize your mistake and have to loop back.

Downloading a map of the trail through an app like AllTrails is a lifesaver. It tracks your progress and lets you know when you're off trail. It also tracks your data and lets you share trail conditions and reviews. Be sure to download the app and the map before you begin, as most trails aren't known for good cell service.

Another option is to take a pic of the map before you start. You'll usually see a detailed map on a guidepost or kiosk near the trailhead.

## Plan for the weather

When you hike is often as important as where you hike. Check the weather for that location a few days ahead of time and right before you go. Sounds pretty obvious, right? Yet it's amazing how many times you see folks on the trail who obviously didn't open a weather app or consult Al Roker before leaving home.

Rainy weather is not only a drag to hike in, it can also turn undeveloped trails into slippery mud slides. Tough to climb and even more dangerous to descend. Not to mention dry creek beds and waterfalls can quickly turn into raging torrents that are treacherous to cross. Freezing cold? You'll want thick layers and gloves and certainly a hat. And never underestimate the digit-saving awesomeness of Hot Hands and Toasti-Toes Toe Warmers. Blazing sun? You'll want a hat, sunscreen, maybe even layers of breathable clothing, especially if you're sun sensitive. Hot and muggy? It'll be sweaty and buggy. Windy days can mean branches down, not to mention pollen all around.

## WELLNESS IN THE WOODS

With all that said, inclement weather can still be a fantastic time to hike. The trails may be less crowded and more exhilarating, as nature flexes.

### STAY SAFE OUT THERE

A good hike is a safe hike. While most day hikes are fairly free of danger, there's always an element of risk. This is wild and wooly nature after all.

As just stated, it's a good idea to check the weather and trail conditions before you head out, and gear up appropriately for the adventure. Be sure to bring plenty of water, nutritious snacks, and any medication you might need if your hike goes longer than expected. Speaking of hikes that go long, it's a good idea to have a flashlight of some kind. The woods get dark quickly when the sun sets and it's easy to get disoriented in the dark. I love the headlamp my daughter got me; it's been a blessing finding my way back to the car. If you're counting on your phone's flashlight, make sure it's fully charged before you head out. It's also smart to let someone know where you are going and when you expect to be back, especially if you're hiking alone.

Pack a small first aid kid in your backpack. I've recently started carrying one in mine. Fortunately I haven't had to use it yet and hopefully never will. But better safe than sorry. You can find great prepacked ones at REI, Amazon, and other retailers.

Each trail comes with its own challenges, so you'll want to be keenly aware of your surroundings. After a few miles it can be easy to let your mind wander and lose focus. But each step matters. Watch for hazards like loose rocks, slippery slopes, fallen branches, rushing waters, exposed tree roots (I've tripped on way too many), even wildlife. Of course sometimes your fellow hikers are the biggest hazard of all.

Despite the temptation, stay on the marked trail. Sometimes the views look too good to resist, but the caution signs are there for a reason. This is especially true if you're hiking with children or pets. You'll want to make sure they stay safe and away from potential harm. Many parks have designated pet trails perfect for our canine companions.

## Hiking solo vs. hiking together

This is such a personal choice. Some hikers prefer the solitude of having the trail all to themselves, surrounded by nothing but nature. It's an exhilarating sense of freedom and adventure. You can travel at your own pace and take breaks whenever you feel like it. You're left alone with your thoughts and the sounds of nature — or your favorite playlist.

But other times, you may crave companionship on the trail. There's something special about sharing a new trail or familiar favorite with a hiking partner. It's a great bonding adventure. It's also helpful to have someone with you to get through tough parts of the trail; lending a hand to cross a creek, climb an incline, or shoo away a snake. Yes, that's happened.

If you're just getting started, it's not a bad idea to have a hiking buddy. If you have friends or family members who like to hike, ask if you can join them sometime. More likely than not, they'll be happy to share some tips and introduce you to some of their favorite hikes.

There are also a lot of hiking clubs out there that plan regular outings and welcome new members. REI and other outdoor-focused companies are a good place to start your online search.

My daughter Hannah, a true trail enthusiast, initiated a hiking club at her previous workplace Experience Columbus, the convention and tourism marketing organization for central Ohio. What started as a small group of trail-curious co-workers grew into "Hikes with Hannah," a sanctioned and frequently scheduled health program loved by many and embraced by the firm's leadership. They saw the substantial health benefits and team-building spirit of the afternoon hikes she led. Employees bonded on the trail during work hours, and the organization offered a great perk in the parks.

## Mindfulness vs. music

Most of the time the sounds of nature are the perfect soundtrack for your hike. The wind whistling through the trees, birds chirping their favorite ditties, frogs croaking across the pond, and the scuffle of your steady bootsteps. Often, that's all you need. Finding mindfulness in the moment. But sometimes you want that perfect playlist where the beat grabs your feet, wakes up your ears, and picks up your pace...especially if it's a trail you've traveled before.

What makes the perfect playlist? For me it's mostly rock or reggae or indie or New Wave. Or blues or zydeco or dixieland. Yacht rock? You bet. I love everything from folk to funk, from ska music to spa music.

While I'm always up for listening to something brand new, I do have a few go-to's that get me going on my Hiking Hits playlist:

**"Jamming" by Bob Marley and the Wailers.** This one always puts a smile on my face no matter where I hear it, but especially on the trail. It's from the 1977 album *Exodus*, which Time Magazine dubbed, "Album of the Century." It's that good.

**"Peach Fuzz" by Caamp.** This Ohio-based band sounds like your best friends singing and strumming and rocking out around a warm, welcoming campfire after a hardy hike.

**"One Step Beyond" by Madness.** I realize British ska isn't everyone's cup of...tea. But if you were a ska punk rude boy in the late 70s and early 80s you knew the power of this infectious rhythm. This Madness song (with the perfect title for hiking) never fails to get me skanking on the trail.

**"Rosalita" by Bruce Springsteen.** Is this The Boss' best? For me it is. A youthful shout-along for full-throttled freedom and the promise of an unbridled tomorrow.

**"Forgot about Dre" by Dr. Dre and Eminem.** The back-and-forth with Dre and Em works perfectly, and adds some swagger to your stride when you need it most on an uphill climb.

**"Telephone" by Lady Gaga and Beyonce.** Pick up the phone...and the pace.

**"From a Buick 6" by Bob Dylan.** I love Bob Dylan so much I named my son after him. I explained this to Dylan when he was about 6. We listened to a bunch of his music and the befuddled boy said, "Why didn't you pick someone who could sing?" Despite that review, I still constantly rock to Robert Zimmerman while driving and hiking. Especially the roadhouse blues-y ravers like this one.

**"Texas Sun" by Khruangbin and Leon Bridges.** I suppose you should know how to pronounce an artist's name if you're adding them to your favorites list, but I'm still not sure I know how to say this one. However, I do know that after one listen, you'll put this song on constant repeat.

**"Weekend Vibe" by Jubel.** Deliciously catchy and the perfectly poppy BPM to keep your boots scootin'.

**"Despacito" by Luis Fonsi, Daddy Yankee, Justin Bieber.** I may not be fluent in Spanish, but apparently my hiking boots are. That tempo works every time.

**"You Know My Name" by Chris Cornell.** I've always been a James Bond fan. And now that Sean Connery has been canceled, the best Bond is Daniel

Craig. His performances always balance suave spy sophistication with English bulldog in a china shop athleticism. This track is my favorite Bond theme from my favorite Bond film, *Casino Royale*. Every time I hear it my mind replays the unbelievable freerunning scenes with Craig chasing the bad guy up and down a high-rise construction site, jumping from girder to girder with parkour perfection.

**"57 Chevy" by Stop Light Observations.** My new fave find. A brilliant pop rock outfit from South Carolina. This song stomps, as will your boots when hiking to it.

**"Backatown" by Trombone Shorty.** Funky n' jazzy instrumental from the New Orleans legend.

**"Thunderstruck" by AC/DC.** For five years my ad agency co-workers and I used to do an intense crossfit workout every day at lunch, challenging ourselves and our bodies. The hour grind usually concluded with a hellish "finisher" devised by the devil himself. One of the most grueling — yet oddly addictive — finishers was executed to this song. The entire group gathered in a circle on the turf, high-stepping rapidly in place. Every time AC/DC lead singer Brian Johnson screams "Thun-der" the entire group had to hit the turf and do a burpee. Actually every time he shrieked "Thunder" or "Thunderstruck." If you're familiar with this awesome Aussie band's work, you know that's a lot of Thunders. 34 to be exact. 34 exhausting grass drills without stopping. When I listen to this track on the trail, I think back fondly...and really appreciate that I don't have to do it here.

**"Tears of a Clown" by The English Beat.** A ska raver that reimagines the Smokey Robinson classic. With just the right tempo to tame the trail.

**"On the Road Again" by Willie Nelson.** The perfect song to finish a day of woods wandering, especially when you're back in the car driving home.

Pumped up or chilled out? What's on your perfect playlist?

## Hike Hack: "Roam" wasn't built in a day

If I'm on a treadmill at the gym and max out, I can slow down or hop off. If I'm traipsing on a long walk through the city and get tired (or even worse, a blister), Uber to the rescue. But if I gas out six miles into a 12 mile hike that finishes with a steep uphill, that's another story. So if you're new to hiking, it's a good idea to start with shorter, easier hikes before attempting more challenging ones. Build up your legs and lungs over time. It's ok to start slowly and gradually increase the distance and difficulty of your adventures.

DAVID HENTHORNE

## "I WALK SLOWLY, BUT I NEVER WALK BACKWARDS."

— ABRAHAM LINCOLN

Honest Abe dropped some truth with this one. It's a philosophy that speaks to steady progress and determination. It's not always about how fast we go, as long as we keep moving forward.

CHAPTER 7

# Gear up for adventure!

*What to pack in that backpack*

I love Jim Gaffigan. Anyone who can do 15 minutes of Hot Pocket jokes is a national treasure. He also has quite a lot of funny things to say about the absurdity of hiking, and specialized hiking clothes.

But after a ten mile slog through the woods, you'll be glad you've got the right gear, no matter what Jim says.

There are endless options and opinions on what hiking gear to get and where to get it. Google "Hiking Gear" and you'll be served ads from outdoor stores, sporting goods stores, Amazon, Ebay, and a gazillion other websites. In my opinion you don't need the latest and greatest (and most expensive) hiking gear, especially when you're starting out. This is especially true if you're day-hiking 3-13 miles versus longer through-hikes and overnight backpacking. That's a different scenario and requires more intense equipment and thoughtful preparation. REI and Public Lands have trained experts ready and waiting to answer every question you could possibly ask.

With that said, you will still be exercising for hours at a time and want quality gear that fits right, feels comfortable, and keeps you safe. Here are a few suggestions based on me learning the hard way.

### HIKING BOOTS

What kind of shoes do IT workers wear? "Re-Boots."

That's a bad joke but a true story. My advertising agency's old IT guy had the same advice every time I had a vexing computer issue. He'd lumber up from his basement lair and say with a healthy dose of disdain, "Did you try turning it off and back on?" I'd roll my eyes at his overly simplistic suggestion, and then, just to humor him as he hovered over me, I'd push the on/off button on my laptop. Without fail the Mac would shut down, restart... and be good as new. I was on my way again.

The lesson: Never underestimate the power of a good reboot. Or when it comes to hiking, rebooting with the right boots.

Your boots are your best friends on the trail. The wrong footwear can cause aching feet, blisters, joint pain, back pain, and ruin the outing...and several days after. I've seen a lot of people trying to trek in athletic shoes, casual shoes, even, believe it or not, *flip flops*. Those might be great footwear options at other times, but not out here. They're not built for this. You want, no you NEED, hiking boots that fit and feel right.

For far too long I wore boots that were too small for my size-12 feet. They were decent quality, just a size too small. Not sure if my feet grew or my boots shrank or it was the fact I wore thicker hiking socks, but whatever the reason it was time for an upgrade. Sadly I was more concerned with using what I had and not throwing money at it — a long-ago lesson from my overly frugal father. But it was my bruised toes that paid the price.

Life changed when I got my Timberlands. A birthday present from my girlfriend, they're the most comfortable boots I've ever owned. Waterproof for the win in rain and snow, and when crossing streams. Great tread for gripping without slipping. And they're the perfect mid-hiker height above the ankle for stability, warmth and protection from angry vegetation. You can certainly pay more for high-end hiking boots, but for my money (hers, actually) you won't find a better boot of its kind.

While my Timberland mid-hiker boots are the right call most of the time and for most of the trails, there are certain situations where I prefer a lighter, shorter shoe. Merrell makes a lot of great outdoor footwear, including the Moab 3. They're fantastic all-purpose, all-terrain, waterproof boots with a lower profile that exposes the ankle. I really like them when I'm hiking in the warmer summer months, or a drier climate. These Merrells were perfect for a recent trip to Sedona, Arizona for some dusty desert trails. They have enough heft to handle gravel and sand, but with less weight than the bulkier mid-hiker height. That lighter weight matters after many miles of hot, arid conditions. Another bonus of their smaller size and weight comes when you're packing for a trip in a cramped carry-on. The big boots take up a lot of space while these guys are about the size of an athletic shoe.

The moral of the story? Don't skimp on footwear. Your toes will thank you.

*Pro Tip:* I suggest trying on as many different boots as you can, at a store. While online shopping is super convenient and we all do it, for this old-school soul it's still important to actually try something on before I buy it — without the hassle of sending it back if it ain't right. There are so many brands and fits and styles and they all offer something different. Comfort and stability are the keys. And quality does matter. Higher quality materials make for a better boot. I've heard the average hiking boot should last 500 miles or so, and you'll want to make sure all those miles are comfortable ones. Also, when trying on hiking footwear, keep in mind you'll be wearing thicker socks than normal. Wear hiking socks that day.

## Hiking socks

I never thought I'd spend so much time researching and investigating socks. Socks are socks, right? Not quite. Choosing the right hiking socks can make or break the experience. Trust me, on a multi-mile woods walk you want happy feet.

Yes it's about comfort, but that cozy comfort can vary depending on the day's weather, the time of year, the footwear they're fitting into, and the terrain of the hike itself. A muddy mountain hike is a different ballgame than a desert trek.

Hiking socks should be thick, but not so thick that your foot feels cramped in the boot. The sock should fit snug, but not tight. Because your feet will swell some during the hike. As for height, I prefer a Crew Sock most of the year. Crew socks are tall enough to show a few inches above the top of your hiking boot and — if you're wearing shorts — provide great protection from low level bugs, stinging nettles, poison ivy and other joys of hiking. If you're on a summer hike and the trail has highly overgrown vegetation, thistles, insects, etc., I would opt for a taller sock, mid-calf or higher. Or just, you know, wear pants.

## Trekking poles

Confession: I used to snicker at people I'd pass on the trail who used trekking poles (also called hiking poles). With their swinging arms and awkward gait they looked a bit silly to me. It seemed like they went to REI and got every single thing the salesperson told them they needed. They bought all the gear but after a few climbs I imagined all that stuff would end up in the back of a closet.

I always preferred to hike poleless. If Lewis and Clark didn't need high tech hiking poles, why would I? If I encountered a lot of elevation changes or a ton of vegetation encroaching on the path, I'd just find a fallen tree branch to use as a staff, much like Gandalf wandering through Middle Earth.

Boy was I wrong. I owe each of those pole people an apology because trekking poles are a wonder.

These lightweight little miracles of technology take a lot of strain off your joints and stress off your body. And because you're incorporating your arms and shoulders, you're using more muscle groups rather than relying on only your legs, which can help with lower body soreness. They also help you maintain your balance, especially when hiking through uneven terrain.

I've found they make climbing uphill much easier as you spread your body weight over four touch-points (two feet, two poles) instead of all the weight on your legs. Equally important, they cushion the impact on your knees and other joints when you're descending downhill. And once you get the handle of walking with them, you get into a natural rhythm of swinging arms and legs that increases your speed, even on flat ground. Might sound crazy but it's true.

The type of pole you need depends on the type of hiking you're planning to do and the distance you'll cover. Sorta like golf clubs I guess.

WELLNESS IN THE WOODS

My girlfriend Carie got me a fantastic set of carbon fiber poles from Cascade Mountain Tech. (They make aluminum ones as well.) They're super lightweight which is great during a long hike, but also if you're carrying them in a backpack or packing them for a trip. They also come with a variety of "feet" which can be swapped out depending on the terrain you're hiking through and the weather conditions: icy, snowy, muddy, etc.

*Pro Tip:* Trekking poles are not only great for climbing, descending and balance, they also make a great tool on the trail. Pushing back dense vegetation as you walk, taking down spiderwebs before they hit your face, providing a helping hand as you cross a creek, and once or twice they even helped me shoo a snake off the path. Much better than surprising it with your boot.

## Your backpack has your back

While traveling light is nice, it's even nicer to be prepared for whatever the trail might throw your way. This is especially true if the conditions are iffy. While you don't need a hundred pound backpack loaded with gear, you want to have the essentials for a happy hike.

- **Water, water, water.** Yes, you need lots of water. Even when it's not hot and humid. Staying hydrated is a no-brainer but I've seen too many people go out for a casual hike without any water. If you get lost or things go long you'll be glad you brought the extra bottle(s). Consider a Camelbak backpack that has a refillable bladder connected to a sipping tube. These are especially helpful in extra arid climates.

- **Sunscreen.** My younger self never applied sunscreen unless I was at the beach. Really wish I could get a mulligan on that. I think I bought my dermatologist a house the past few years. While we all love that vitamin D, sun damage is no joke. Experts recommend an SPF of at least 30 or higher, applied to any exposed skin and reapplied often. And while we usually think about sunburn in the warmer months, don't forget to apply sunscreen in winter too. Especially if there's snow on the ground, when the sun's rays can bounce up and do some damage.

- **Bug Spray.** This one is a must. I can't count the times I wish I had brought bug spray to ward off tiny buzzing beasts. So now it's a constant companion, especially on summer hikes or anywhere there's dense vegetation.

- **Headlamp.** This is a new addition to my backpack, thanks to my outdoor-loving daughter. Sometimes the trail goes longer and later than you planned, or you'll discover a cavern waiting to be explored, or you're just in the mood for a pre-dawn adventure.

Whatever the reason, having a headlamp is an easy-to-carry insurance policy for finding your way out.

- **First Aid Kit.** Although you're on a day hike not a cross-country expedition, you'll still want to have a little "Just in Case" kit. They sell pre-packed ones at REI and other places that have the basics covered. It's best to have a kit that includes antiseptic wipes, antibacterial ointment, assorted bandages (for assorted blisters), ibuprofen, bug bite/anti-itch treatment, antihistamine to treat allergic reactions, and of course any medications you might need.

- **Pen and Paper.** You never know when you'll be inspired to release your inner Thoreau or Picasso, write a love note or lively limerick, draw a treasure map or sketch a Sasquatch.

- **Snacks.** Finally the fun part. Packing those snacks! You can burn a lot of calories hiking — an average adult can burn between 300-600 calories per hour depending on terrain, intensity, distance and their own weight. Of course healthier snacks are the best choice when it's time to refuel. There are plenty of hiker-friendly energy bars, granola bars, protein bars, etc. I'm a big fan of bananas, apples, almonds, peanut butter and beef jerky. Of course we're assuming you ate a good meal before hitting the trail so you have a good base and don't get light-headed along the way. Pack whatever snacks (or meals even) make sense, and that you'll actually eat. Basically, don't hike on an empty stomach, nobody wants a hangry hiker wandering the woods.

## Cold weather gear

Don't underestimate the wonder of a cold-weather hike. It can be beautiful and a totally different trail than in warmer months. But also don't underestimate the extra challenges it presents. It's about comfort, but also safety.

The best advice is to dress in layers. Most experts recommend a three-part system to keep Mother Nature off your back. A base layer to wick away perspiration, a mid layer that insulates to keep you warm, and an outer shell layer to keep wind and moisture out. Layering lets you adjust for comfort and changing conditions throughout your hike. When you've heated up remove a layer; when you're cold add it back. The ultimate goal is to stay dry and avoid hypothermia.

It's equally important to avoid frostbite on exposed skin, such as your face, ears, fingers and toes. Make sure you have good gloves (I prefer them thick but not too thick, this isn't skiing), and a hat that covers your ears and forehead. Warm socks are a must, but if they're too thick they can make your boots too tight and make your feet uncomfortable. Wool or synthetic are your best options. Always a good idea to bring an extra pair, in case they get wet. Hiking with wet feet is no bueno.

If you're sensitive to cold fingers and toes, Hot Hands and Toe Warmers packets are your best bets on the trail. Don't forget these small but mighty digit savers.

Maybe the best cold weather tip of all is to invest in some Yaktrax. These little marvels are cleats that fit on the bottom of your boots and provide instant traction. They grip the ice and packed snow for extra safety, which is especially helpful when you're hiking on challenging terrain with elevation changes.

## *Hike Hack: 1 trail, 4 seasons*

The brain craves variety. Mine does anyway. But it's nearly impossible to hike a different route every single time. Especially after years of hitting up your local faves as often as possible. One of my favorite ways to feed that need for variety is to hike the same trail during each of the four seasons. Here in the Midwest the seasons change substantially, and each one has its own beauty and impact on nature.

It might seem obvious, but the change of seasons brings big changes to the trail — and your appreciation for it. Spring is an adrenaline rush of new life as the understory wakes from its winter slumber and the trees share their blossoms and buds. Summer hiking is an intense workout with increased heat and humidity, and an obstacle course of overgrown vegetation and buzzing bugs. Fall is like the cool-down after that summer workout, a chance for reconnection and reflection as autumn colors drape the landscape. And don't hibernate on the benefits and beauty of winter hiking. Ice and snow will transform your familiar trail into a winter wanderland, turning waterfalls into icicles so impressive they'd make the North Pole jealous.

What's your most treasured trail? Have you hiked it in all four seasons, or in different weather conditions? It's a great way to find a new adventure on an old favorite.

# "It's not the mountain we conquer, but ourselves."

— Sir Edmund Hillary

CHAPTER 8

# To all the trails I've loved before

*Trails worth trying in this world of wanders*

As we saw in Chapter 1, there are hundreds of thousands of trails worldwide. AllTrails features over 400,000 of them, in 150 countries. Just about anywhere in the world, there's a woods walk waiting to be explored.

Over the years, hiking has become a central consideration while planning upcoming vacations and getaways. Where in the world is our next hike? Who knows, but we almost always create trips around the proximity to interesting new trails. I've also been fortunate to have a career that has let me explore faraway places, from meeting and filming mountain gorillas in Rwanda to hiking the California coast to bungee jumping in New Zealand. Any time a work trip that can include trail time, I'm all in.

## Geology rocks.
## But geography is where it's at.

This passion of mine has taken me to trails on five continents, over 30 U.S. states, and nearly 60 of Ohio's 76 state parks. Whether it's a quick scenic stop or a longer slog, all the trails shared here hold a special place for me, and I hope they will for you too. You can find more information on these hikes and many other adventures on my travel website, WorldOfWanders.com.

   A word of caution: Most of these hikes are popular because they offer some stunning scenery, challenging terrain and a wonderful sense of accomplishment when you reach the summit or complete the trail. But as always, please proceed carefully. Some of these trails can be difficult and even dangerous, so it's important to be prepared, wear the right gear, hike with caution, and bring plenty of water.

## HOCKING HILLS STATE PARK, LOGAN, OHIO
### A state park with national park swagger

## WELLNESS IN THE WOODS

My native Ohio has 76 state parks, and they all have something special about them. From Lake Erie to the Ohio River they are all gems in their own right. But perhaps the shiniest gem of all is Hocking Hills State Park in Logan. Don't just take my word for it. It was recently named "One of the most beautiful state parks" in America, and has been recognized as one of the nation's 50 Best State Parks. Indeed, there are world-class wonders waiting to be discovered in Ohio's Hocking Hills.

The much-loved park is within the iconic Hocking Hills region, and features over 25 miles of world-class hiking trails, Insta-worthy waterfalls, scenic rock formations, cliffs, and caves. All that natural beauty means it's very popular, and can get really crowded during the summer and especially on weekends. Locals flock here, and as you walk through the parking lot you'll see tons of out-of-state plates.

"Hiking" is almost in the name itself. I can't tell you how many times my mouth's worked faster than my brain and I've said, "Hiking Hills." Oh, and you will be. There are plenty of hills to hike, cliffs to climb and trails to tramp. Old Man's Cave gets most of the love, but don't miss out on the roar of Cedar Falls, the massive Ash Cave, the mysterious Rock House, the views at Cantwell Cliffs, and Conkle's Hollow, one of the deepest gorges in Ohio.

**Everybody loves Grandma.** The most popular path is the Grandma Gatewood Trail, starting at the Visitor Center near the Upper Falls and winding its way to the Lower Falls and the fabled Old Man's Cave. Before starting your hike, spend some time at the recently-renovated visitor center discovering plenty of fun facts on the history, topography and wildlife of the area.

As you descend the stairs into the gorge, be sure to look for "The Whale in the Wall." Years ago a friendly ranger pointed it out while my son and I began the trail. Once you see it, you'll never unsee it. A large coloration in the sandstone cliff in the exact shape of a sperm whale, its tail flukes waving and welcoming you.

Look for the Grandma Gatewood trail signs. The trail is named after Emma Rowena Caldwelll Gatewood, a Hocking Hills trailblazer born in 1887 and the first woman to solo hike the Appalachian Trail.

It's a beautiful but often challenging 3-mile hike from the visitor center to Cedar Falls, then another 3 miles to the breathtaking Ash Cave. You'll encounter the Upper Falls, the Lower Falls, Devil's Bathtub, the Sphinx, plenty of bouldering, a million tree roots trying to trip you, and more photo ops than you can shake your iPhone at. It's 12 miles round-trip so bring trail snacks and lots of water.

*Pro tip:* Hiking the trails when crowds aren't is much more enjoyable. We once did a fantastic Friday late afternoon/early evening hike and had the park almost to ourselves. Some afternoon rain added to the magic as the waterfalls were flexing and pouring it on.

**Warm up to winter hiking.** While Hocking

Hills State Park is most popular in the warmer months, don't shy away from a winter wander. Not only is it less crowded, it also takes on an icy Game of Thrones north-of-the-Wall vibe. The cliffs and waterfalls show off colossal icicle formations and the rushing creeks gurgle beneath the slippery surface. Plus the crowds are one tenth the size. Be warned, it gets extremely icy and the falls can be perilous. Dress warmly and wear Yak Tracks or other traction cleats.

## VOLCANOES NATIONAL PARK, RWANDA
### Rwanda wandering: Meeting mountain gorillas in Africa

A fully-grown male silverback gorilla can weigh around 400 pounds. They're also 6 to 9 times stronger than a full-grown human. So coming face-to-face with one on their turf can be hella intimidating. Meeting mountain gorillas in the wild is also one of the most memorable, adrenalin-fueled experiences on Earth.

Our adventure began while filming in northwest Rwanda, in Volcanoes National Park. Located in a truly remote rainforest, the park is nestled in the Virunga Mountains conservation region. This isn't your everyday hike through a city park; it's a challenging multi-mile slog up and down steep mountains, along muddy barely-there paths through thick primordial jungle filled with stinging nettles and thorny plants. It ain't easy. Fortunately, the local guides are helpful and patient. Tourism is vital to the local economy, as is the survival of the mountain gorillas that are so revered.

After a week's safari filming in nearby Kenya, this part of Africa feels a million miles away. It's a different kind of beautiful here. Green and lush and filled with life — and unusual sounds of life. Odd birds squawking overhead, hungry bugs buzzing in your ears, the clapping of our lead guide to warn snakes and other creepy crawlies of our approach. Every time something scuttles through the underbrush you wonder what you'd see in there...and what might be watching you.

Part of our trek takes us to the tomb of Dian Fossey, the respected American primatologist and conservationist. She became world-famous for studying mountain gorilla groups extensively from 1966 until her murder in 1985. She documented their behaviors, lived among them, and became their greatest champion.

**Gorillas reign in the rainforest.** Hours into our journey over slippery slopes and through multiple pop-up showers, we enter a clearing and can't believe our eyes. There they are, wondrous and wild and free. A troop of majestic mountain gorillas. Foraging and frolicking. Staring back at us. Not afraid of us, just...observing us. The main silverback is truly massive. This is the true King of the Jungle. A hulking beast, yet gentle as can be with the young ones climbing all over him. We're just thankful they're plant-eaters.

We wander among them for some time, quietly filming, photographing and respecting them and their home. Just two species not that far apart evolutionarily speaking. In fact, data confirms that humans and gorillas are about 98 percent identical on a genetic level. In this moment, in this rainforest, watching gorilla mothers and fathers and children interact and share a meal, that feels about right.

The nearest airport to Volcanoes National Park in Rwanda is Kigali International Airport in Kigali, Rwanda's capital city. It's a 3-hour drive from Kigali to Volcanoes National Park, where hiking expeditions begin. Gorilla Trek Permits must be purchased through the official government website or from licensed tour operators.

## POINT PELEE NATIONAL PARK, ONTARIO
### HIKING CANADA'S SOUTHERNMOST POINT

As a life-long Ohioan I've visited the shores of Lake Erie countless times. Sandusky and Cedar Point and Put-in-Bay and Toledo and Cleveland. But those are the *southern* shores of that Great Lake. I'd never seen Erie looking down from the north. Until now.

Although it feels a world away, this part of Canada is just a four-hour drive from Columbus. We found a charming AirBnB right on the water near

Leamington, Ontario. It had the total relaxey vibe and nautical themed decor you want on a beach town getaway. The dogs were mesmerized by the raging waves and crashing surf right in the backyard. The small local beach was just a five minute walk...which Oscar the Boston Terrier insisted on twice a day. We told him it was the ocean and he seemed to buy it.

The highlight of the trip was a visit to "the Tip of Canada," Point Pelee National Park. Long-ago glaciers and the currents of Lake Erie have created a triangular spit of land extending nine miles into the lake. It's remarkable to walk out to this southern tip of the country as it narrows and eventually disappears into the waves. And what an effect that thin peninsula has: The waters on the east side of the peninsula are quite choppy, while the waters on the west are as calm as the Caribbean.

Point Pelee National Park features miles of interesting trails through forests and beaches and boardwalks, plus there's a ton of cool local history to discover. Plan to spend a day, there's that much to see and do.

## DEVIL'S BRIDGE/WEST FORK, ARIZONA
### RED ROCKS, RAD TRAILS IN SEDONA

Sedona is just a short and beautiful 2-hour drive from Phoenix. The popular tourist town has been called a cathedral without walls, and after spending a few days there now I know why. As you approach the town it feels sacred, as if mysterious forces are emanating from those red rocks. People come here from all over the world for the mystical vortexes and natural healing powers. My buddies and I found our own nirvana in Sedona playing golf, riding ATVs, telling old jokes, and especially while hiking.

**West Fork Trail.** The popular West Fork Trail is a sweet 6-mile hike with amazing views as you wind your way through the cliffs and canyons in Coconino National Forest. It helps to download AllTrails as there are plenty of overlapping trails that intersect. There's parking and restrooms at the trailhead. The views are sensational, especially early or late in the day (it's also way easier to get a parking spot then).

I didn't think that hike could be topped, but the final hike of our visit changed my mind. Surprisingly, I hadn't even heard of Devil's Bridge or seen photos of it. Which honestly made it that much more spectacular when we arrived at the summit.

**"Built by the Devil himself"** The Devil's Bridge Trail is six miles roundtrip from the parking area and one of the greatest hikes you'll ever do, leading to a breathtaking, daredevil, "don't look down," Instagrammable moment you'll cherish forever. The bridge itself is the largest natural sandstone arch in the Sedona area. According to legend it was built by ol' Beelzebub, as no mortals could construct anything so difficult. Despite its name, it's one of the mostly heavenly things you'll ever see.

It's spectacular just to see the arch and the canyon behind it. But the real thrill comes walking out across it, which the brave certainly do. It's a photo opp you won't want to miss, and fellow hikers are usually happy to take your pic out on the bridge if you return the favor. Fortunately, I gave my camera to a young European tourist who knew how to take pictures and capture the moment, as my buddy is terrible at it.

*Pro tip:* If you can time your hike so you get there around sunset, the light in the canyon is perfect. And no joke, bring water. Lots of it.

## CLEAR CREEK METRO PARK, OHIO
### THIS AIN'T YOUR AVERAGE WALK IN THE PARK

One of the most challenging — and beautiful — hikes in the Midwest can be found at Clear Creek Metro Park, about 45 minutes southeast of Columbus in the foothills of the Appalachians. It's a big park, with over 5400 acres of wooded wilderness and 15 miles of scenic trails.

You know you're someplace special as soon as you enter the park, as a massive leaning boulder appears to block the road itself. It goes by many names: Leaning Rock, Leaning Lena, even Witches Rock. That last nickname comes from an urban legend of witches gathering nearby, especially at Halloween.

There's a rich history here. Indigenous people were the original settlers long ago. Later, Europeans arrived and evidence of their agriculture and industry remain, with abandoned mills and cemeteries throughout the park.

One of the main trails takes its spooky name from a graveyard. The difficult Cemetery Ridge is only 2.5 miles but the initial climb is insanely steep and will knock your lungs for a loop. It's not for the faint of heart. However, you will be rewarded along the way with a peek at the stunning Yellow Lady's Slipper orchid. The Chestnut, Fern and Hemlock trails are all lovely to look at — and laborious to conquer with their up and down elevations. Near the Lake trail be on the lookout for the telltale gnawings of beavers.

## PATH OF THE GODS, AMALFI COAST, ITALY
### A HEAVENLY HIKE ON ITALY'S PATH OF THE GODS

Some hikes stay with you forever. This most definitely is one of them.

I've been fortunate to visit Italy a few times, but never had I been to the postcard-perfect town of Positano on the Amalfi Coast. A jewel of southern Italy, this area is known for its dramatic cliffs, turquoise waters, breathtaking scenery, and colorful towns clinging to the rugged coastline. As if that weren't enough, high above Positano waits one of the world's great hikes.

DAVID HENTHORNE

**"Sentiero degli Dei"** Path of the Gods ("Sentiero degli Dei") is a legendary 4.5 mile trail with unparalleled views, a rich history, and plenty of Mediterranean magic. The path hugs the cliffs at the dizzying height of 2065 feet above sea level. While we were excited to explore Positano, nearby Sorrento, Pompeii and other area sights, this hike was a big reason for our Amalfi adventure.

Legends abound regarding the trail's origin. Some say it was built by the ancient Romans as a trade route, while others claim it served as a pathway for Greek gods traversing between Mount Olympus and their earthly domains. Or, it's a really beautiful goat path with an amazing PR backstory. Regardless of its origin, the Path of the Gods has served as a crucial connection between coastal villages for centuries.

We discovered that if you're staying in Positano, the ideal itinerary is to catch a bus to Bomerano and hike the trail back toward Positano. This way the views are always in front of you, and you finish with the 1700 stair descent back into town. But on this chilly and rainy mid-December day, with intermittent bus service, the odds and the gods were not in our favor.

So we took a local bus from Positano up, up, up to Nocelle, a charming little village high above Positano. Fueling up before the hike, we stopped in an absolutely adorable deli—or, in Italian, "salumeria" which sounds way sexier—for the world's greatest salami and provolone sandwich. While the deli owner spoke no English, she understood exactly what we needed to pregame for the Path of the Gods.

**So many selfies.** The sun played peek-a-boo through the clouds as we spent the next few hours wandering the trail, stopping every few seconds to take in the view, take photos, and utter "Wow" endlessly. The views truly are breathtaking, and there are unexpected delights along the way, including several ancient ruins to explore. While the weather was less than ideal, on the plus side our December hike meant we had the trail almost completely to ourselves. We saw maybe half a dozen people the entire time. Sounds like that's not the case in warmer months, when crowds overtake the path. It's worth considering planning your visit during a less crowded off-season time.

"Sentiero degli Dei" is more than just another hike. It's an epic journey for the soul. It feels timeless, as you're surrounded by ageless cliffs, Old World culture and the mythical Mediterranean.

*Pro tip:* The Path of the Gods is a moderately difficult hike with some uneven terrain, loose rocks and decent inclines. We're glad we brought our hiking shoes. Bring water in that backpack, there aren't places to stop along the way. Shade is limited on the trail, so sunscreen is a good idea too, even in the cooler months like our December trek.

DAVID HENTHORNE

## SEQUOIA AND KINGS CANYON, CALIFORNIA
### NATIONAL PARKS WITH NATIONAL TREASURES

A few years ago I had a travel dilemma. I had just finished a week filming commercials in Los Angeles, and had a meeting in San Francisco on Monday. Should I fly all the way across the country to be back in Ohio for a split second, or spend those days hiking two of America's most spectacular national parks? When would I have a chance like this again?

A quick Google search helped me make up my mind. Sequoia National Park is about 200 miles north of Los Angeles and 260 miles east of San Francisco, in the beautiful southern Sierra Nevada mountains. Plus it's a 2-for-1, as Kings Canyon National Park is right next door. (As I discovered, "right next door" means something different with our massive national parks; it was a colossal commute between the two.) I rented a car and started the drive from Santa Monica to Sequoia, excited for the opportunity to hike among the largest living things on Earth.

A few hours in, I saw the sign for Bakersfield, California. I've been a fan of "The Bakersfield Sound" for years. It's a type of country music born in the 1950s right there in that modest little town in the middle of the Golden State. Known for its combo of rock n' roll and honky-tonk, with a healthy dose of backbeats, the Bakersfield Sound was made famous by Buck Owens, Merle Haggard, and my favorite, Dwight Yoakam. As I drove to and through Bakersfield I cranked up some Dwight and motored on toward the mountains.

**Wandering amongst giants.** Established in 1890, Sequoia National Park was created to protect these ancient forests from logging. It's a testament to conservation efforts then (thank you John Muir) and efforts that continue today. One wander through these woods and you'll appreciate the importance of preserving our natural wonders.

I arrived late Friday afternoon at the park entrance, with just a few hours of daylight left. But it was a great appetizer for my Saturday hikes. I was able to stretch my legs and stare up (and up and up) at these magnificent giants while I explored a few of the park's world-famous trails.

First up, I had to see the biggest rock star celebrity of them all. The monster of the forest. The colossal conifer. The world's largest living tree: The General Sherman. The General Sherman Trail is an easy 1.2 miles, but when you're here it's not about length, it's about height. And weight. And width. That's what makes the General Sherman the biggest on Earth. No other tree has the combined weight and width of this multi-limbed leviathan. It's estimated to be 1,385 tons, 103 feet around, 275 feet high — and still growing. In fact, every year the old General (estimated to be over 2,500 years old) adds enough wood to make another 60-foot-tall tree. Mind blown yet? How about this? One branch of this tree is so enormous, a whopping 7 feet in diameter, that it's larger than most trees in the Eastern U.S.

DAVID HENTHORNE

So yeah, it's big.

Near the General Sherman Trail is the Congress Trail, an easy 2-mile loop that weaves and winds through towering sequoia groves and meadows, with some truly stunning views. I marveled at plenty of other titans of the forest as the sun set and the temperature dropped.

Saturday morning, fueled by an almost adequate free hotel breakfast and the promise of more giant sightings, I headed back to Sequoia. My first stop was the Giant Forest Museum. It's a great way to learn about the history, geography and ecology of the park, with lots of cool interactive exhibits. The adjacent Big Trees Trail is not long but it is stunning, with educational trailside panels as you learn about the sequoias up close.

I had heard good things about the Little Baldy Trail and made that my next hike. The 3.3 mile out-and-back trail climbs along a meandering network of switchbacks to the top of a granite dome, with plenty of native wildflowers and ferns along the way. It's listed as "moderately challenging" on AllTrails, with an 800-foot elevation gain, but it felt more strenuous than that being so high up in the mountains. While the views are said to be awesome, on this day it was cloudy and socked in, so I had to imagine the vistas below. What I also had to do was record a video message at the top of "Little Baldy" to my younger brother Chris, who happens to be a Little Baldy himself.

WELLNESS IN THE WOODS

I explored a few other trails that afternoon as the weather turned wilder, before heading back to the warmth of the hotel.

*Pro Tip:* If you're visiting Sequoia, do yourself a favor and spend some time at the awesome Three Rivers Brewing. It was right by my hotel just outside the gateway to the national park, in the village of Three Rivers. They have great beer, friendly people, and even live music around a campfire. What a happy, hoppy way to wind down your adventure.

**The king of Kings Canyon.** On the last day of my micro-adventure, I headed to the adjacent (but still took a while to get to) Kings Canyon National Park. This park is no slouch either when it comes to huge redwood trees. They're everywhere. The big boy in this park is the famous General Grant tree, located in the tongue-twistery General Grant Grove. Not only is it the 2nd-largest tree in the world, it's also affectionately nicknamed "The Nation's Christmas Tree." Good luck putting a star on top of that one.

I wandered a few amazing trails around the giants before heading to the park's other masterpiece, Cedar Grove. With its towering cliffs and cascading waterfalls it's breathtaking in its own right. So much so that John Muir once called this part of Kings Canyon, "a rival to Yosemite." He oughta know.

**Tips for visiting Sequoia & Kings Canyon.** It's best to plan ahead (unlike I did). As I had to schedule on the day of my arrival, I was lucky to get the last room at a small hotel just outside the park. Accommodations throughout the area and parking lots inside the parks fill up quickly, especially during peak season.

Be sure to dress in layers. The park's elevation ranges from 6,000 to 8,000 feet, so temperatures can vary greatly depending on time of day and the trail you're on. They sure did for me. Also, at that elevation you're often hiking through the clouds themselves, so it can be misty and damp.

Bring water and snacks. You're there for the remoteness and connection with nature, but that also means there aren't convenience stores loaded with goodies every quarter mile. Plan ahead and pack that backpack.

## RED RIVER GORGE, KENTUCKY
### AMAZING TRAILS NEAR THE BOURBON TRAIL

Some of the best hiking in the Eastern U.S. can be found just an hour east of Lexington, Kentucky. The Red River Gorge Geological Area is a huge 29,000-acre area nestled in the rustic Daniel Boone National Forest. According to travel websites, the Red River Gorge is the "Adventure Capital of Kentucky," and has amazed visitors ever since Boone himself first set foot here in the late 1700s. It amazed us too.

Based on recommendations from friends and All-Trails, we chose the Auxier Ridge Trail to Courthouse Rock, a 4.5-mile out-and-back trek with amazing views of the gorge below. It earned every bit of its "moderately challenging" rating. Lots of elevation changes. It reminded us of the challenging trails and rock formations at Ohio's Airplane Rock, one of our favorite hikes. There were tons of other outdoor lovers on the trail, including many four-legged ones with wagging tails. We got slobbered on a lot. As if that wasn't enough hiking for the day, we also climbed to the top of nearby Natural Bridge State Park, named after an amazing natural sandstone arch spanning 78 feet and standing over 65 feet high. The climb was rough but the view from the arch was totally worth it. Highly recommended. 10 out of 10, would do it again.

We can't wait to go back to Kentucky, where bluegrass and bourbon rule and the gorges are gorgeous.

*Pro tip:* If you're in the Red River Gorge area, be sure to stop at Miguel's Pizza, a hip pizza cafe plus climbing gear shop and campground. The pizza is fantastic, hits the spot after a day on the trails, and the rock climbing crowd gives the joint some lively, outdoorsy energy.

## NEUSCHWANSTEIN CASTLE, GERMANY
**Fairy-tale trails in Bavaria**

## DAVID HENTHORNE

Once upon a time in a land far, far away, a father and his young son wandered an enchanted forest in the shadows of a storybook castle.

It's not a fairy tale, it was a true trail tale for Dylan and me, in the Bavarian region of Germany. Neuschwanstein Castle towers over the landscape of southern Germany near the Austrian border in the foothills of the Alps. Not only is this awe-inspiring palace one of the top tourist attractions in Bavaria, it's also the real-life inspiration for Cinderella's Castle at Disneyland. It's easy to see how Walt took one look and said, "Yep, that's it."

It's an easy and enjoyable two-hour train ride from Munich to Füssen. Europeans certainly know how to do rail right. Can't wait until passenger train travel becomes more common and appreciated in the U.S. From the train station it's a ten minute bus ride to Schwangau where the castle is located, or you can challenge yourself with the uphill walk to the gates. The elevation is a bit intense.

While the tour inside the 65,000 square-foot castle is an epic must-see, so are the trails that surround the estate. Considered moderately challenging, the 4.3-mile out-and-back trail offers a totally different perspective of Neuschwanstein and its idyllic countryside. The first part of the trail has a lot of tourists but it becomes less crowded as you continue on. Watch out for plenty of exposed tree roots trying to trip you. The big reward awaits you at the bridge: absolutely stunning views of Neuschwanstein Castle and the green valley below.

No wonder Walt was inspired by this magical palace, and magical place.

## MOONVILLE TUNNEL, OHIO
### A HAUNTED HIKE WITH A GHOST TRAIN TRAIL

Legend has it there's a haunted railroad tunnel in Vinton County, Ohio. So of course we had to walk through it at night. On Halloween. Now dotted with graffiti and loaded with haunted hype, Moonville Tunnel strikes an imposing image as you approach. Moonville was a small mining and railway town that popped up during the 1800s iron boom, yet totally disappeared years later. Barely a trace left behind.

According to local legend, the host ghost is that of a railroad worker who was crushed by an oncoming train in the spring of 1859. Those who claim to have seen him say he carries a lantern and often appears as a hovering orb of light. Others say the tunnel is haunted by the ghost of a pregnant woman struck by a train. Four other souls were reportedly killed at the tunnel as well.

Whatever you believe, you can definitely feel a macabre sense of mystery as you approach the tunnel's gaping maw. Not gonna lie, it's pretty spooky. Especially after a 10-mile hike on Halloween night went longer than expected, forcing us to walk back through the empty tunnel in the pitch black of a chilly and chilling late October night. Your footsteps seem to echo louder in the dark, and the dim light at the end of the tunnel feels impossibly far away. Yikes.

Fortunately, the area surrounding the Moonville Tunnel is gorgeous, lush...and filled with life. Nearby Lake Hope State Park and Zaleski State Forest are loaded with amazing hiking trails. Some of the best in Ohio. And Moonville is just a 30-minute drive from the natural wonders of the popular Hocking Hills region. The history and biodiversity of the area are spectacular and well worth witnessing.

Just keep your ears open for the haunted whistle of a ghost train echoing in the distance.

## **ACADIA NATIONAL PARK, MAINE**
### **HIKING THE ROCKY COAST OF MAINE**

I've always been fascinated with Maine. The remoteness, the accent, the lobsters. It always seemed like the "wildest" of the eastern states. While I'd been to New England plenty of times, I'd never ventured that far northeast. Until a work trip filming commercials took me to Bar Harbor, Maine, a terrific tourist town bustling with cinematic East Coast charm.

Fortunately, it's also right next door to Acadia National Park. Unfortunately, I only had a few hours to explore it. But what fun it was packing trail time into those too few minutes.

At 1532 feet, Acadia's famous Cadillac Mountain is the highest point along the North Atlantic

# WELLNESS IN THE WOODS

seaboard, giving visitors a panoramic perspective of the world below. The Great Head Trail is a quick 1.9 miles roundtrip, but offers plenty of ocean views and rocky scrambles. The trailhead starts at Sand Beach, which is a picturesque pitstop and great selfie location.

There are over 150 miles of hiking trails in Acadia, in so many environments from mountaintops to spruce-fir forests to seashore. And I got to explore so few of them. The views are spectacular in every direction and you'll be gobsmacked no matter which way you look. I sure was. Can't wait to visit again, hike more trails...and try more lobster rolls.

### WHAT ARE YOUR 3 FAVORITE TRAILS ANYWHERE IN THE WORLD?

Mt. Fuji summit trail, The Cinque Terre trail, and any trail around Crested Butte, Colorado during the peak wildflower season in early July.  **– Scott, Colorado**

1) Grotto Falls in the Smoky Mountains. It's an easy hike with a big payoff!
2) Kamama Prairie, Arc of Appalachia. Stun-

ning biodiversity that includes butterflies and prairie flowers that are not found in many other places on Earth.
3) Horseshoe Falls at Caesar Creek. A wonderful hike through deep woods and a destination that includes the falls and a swing bridge over the river.
**– Lisa, Ohio**


1) Strouds Run State Park, Athens, Ohio. I trained for triathlons and 50ks on these trails. The memories of training there during the gray winter months, then driving into Athens to visit my brother at Ohio University, are some of my fondest.
2) Lake Solitude, Grand Teton National Park, Wyoming. For a day hike, this trail is a doozy. With over 2300 feet of elevation gain, the glutes are burning by the time you reach the pristine blue alpine lake. The icy jump into the water is one of the most refreshing experiences of my life. Along the way, wildflowers, moose, and babbling brooks line the trail.
3) Lamar Valley, Yellowstone National Park, Wyoming. One of my favorite movies growing up was the animated movie about dinosaurs, The Land Before Time. Lamar Valley takes up the easternmost section of the mammoth-sized Yellowstone National Park,

and it is that movie brought to life. Except now, instead of dinosaurs, bison roam these verdant plains.
**– Hannah, Colorado**


1) Wildwood Trail in Portland because of its nearness and familiarity.
2) The hike in and out of the Grand Canyon due to the surroundings and the feeling you've accomplished something that's bucket-list worthy.
3) Sunset Peak in Hong Kong – Challenging and an amazing view.
**– John, Oregon**

## RED ROCK CANYON, NEVADA
### VIVA LAS RED ROCKS!

Red Rock Canyon National Conservation Area is just 19 minutes from the Las Vegas Strip, but feels a world away. The only bright lights here are the stars in the clear skies at night.

I've been to this Mojave Desert wonderland a few times, and always leave in awe. The canyon is an area of global geologic interest, with its towering sandstone and limestone peaks (some reaching 7,000 feet!), 26 robust hiking trails, and vivid colors that live up to the Red Rock name.

The headliner at this near-Vegas showcase is the one-way 13-mile scenic drive, which gives you access to plenty of spectacular overlooks and local history. Be sure to stop at the visitor center inside the main gate for helpful information and trail maps.

My first and favorite hike at Red Rocks Canyon was the Calico Tanks Trail, which is considered one of the most popular in the park. The trailhead can be found at the Sandstone Quarry parking lot. How did it get such an unusual name? "Calico" because of the alternate red and white markings in the rock formations, and "Tanks" because you'll pass pocket tanks that fill with rainwater at certain times of the year. It's 2.4 miles and ranked moderate to strenuous in difficulty. There's a good deal of boulder scrambling and elevation so be prepared. Also, it's hot. Way hot. Bring plenty of water, more than you might think. The reward at the end of the out-and-back mountain trail is a stunning aerial view of Sin City like you've never seen it, sitting in the distant desert. You can almost hear Wayne Newton from here.

I hiked a few more miles on a few other epic trails, and made a couple scenic stops at the High Point Overlook and the Red Rock Wash Overlook. Even if you're not up for hiking or feeling the heat, that 13-mile drive is worth the trip.

## WELLNESS IN THE WOODS

### CHRISTMAS ROCKS NATURE AREA, OHIO
#### GIFTS ARE WAITING AT CHRISTMAS ROCKS

The name sounds like a bebopping Brenda Lee holiday classic, but Christmas Rocks is actually a gorgeous and challenging hike in the Appalachian foothills. Best of all, there's a big gift waiting at the top of its famous overlook: a breathtaking view of the Clearcreek Valley nearly 300 feet below. It's a selfie stick paradise.

At this remote, 415-acre heavily wooded preserve you'll find 4.5 miles of hiking trails on two separate loops. To get to the scenic vista at the top of the black hand sandstone cliff, you'll have to conquer the absolutely demonic Jacob's Ladder. I say demonic because the elevation will get your heart pumping, your lungs gasping, and your mouth cursing. But once you've reached the top the view makes it all worthwhile.

The parking lot near the trailhead is small and can fill up quickly on weekends. Near the parking lot, be sure to check out a very cool historic covered bridge, the Mink Hollow Covered Bridge, built in 1887.

### MCKINNEY FALLS/BARTON CREEK, AUSTIN
#### 5-STAR HIKING IN THE LONE STAR STATE

## DAVID HENTHORNE

They say "Everything's bigger in Texas" — and that includes the wonders worth wandering. Exploring Austin offers all kinds of big-time adventures, from cowboy boots to hiking boots.

With its distinct climate, plants, and topography Texas offers some great trails. Just 13 miles from downtown Austin I found the idyllic playground that is McKinney Falls State Park. The rushing waters of Onion Creek have carved breathtaking grooves into the ancient limestone, creating an otherworldly terrain. A variety of trails wind their way through scenic Hill Country woods and historic sights to the Upper Falls and Lower Falls. It's truly breathtaking.

**No waterfalls? No problem.** Located in south-central Austin, the Barton Creek Greenbelt Trail is 13 miles of hiker's heaven. Considered one of the top hiking trails in Texas, the out-and-back route runs along Barton Creek, which was dry when I visited. So, while there were no waterfalls, the lack of water revealed stunning secrets below. Much like McKinney Falls, the rushing waters have created deep patterns in the limestone creek bed. And they're amazing. Note: I found the trailheads and parking to be a bit confusing (maybe it's just me) so plan accordingly when planning a visit.

One last thing, after that challenging Greenbelt hike I returned to my rental SUV and a tiny shiny something on the ground caught my eye. It was a piece of black glass, somehow in the EXACT shape of the state of Ohio. Thanks for the hospitality

Texas, I guess it's time to go home. Happy hiking, y'all.

## ANTELOPE CANYON/HORSESHOE BEND, AZ
### Wander these real-life screensavers

You know the stunning screensaver photos that pop up every time you ignore your TV for more than a minute? Ever walked through one? You can, at Arizona's Antelope Canyon and Horseshoe Bend.

While on a weekend trip to Sedona, my friends and I took the 3-hour drive north to Page, Arizona. Located just outside Page within the Navajo Nation, Antelope Canyon is unlike any place else. The Navajo Sandstone was formed by deposits swept there by swirling wind 180 million years ago, during the Jurassic Period (sadly we saw no dinosaurs). The breathtaking slot canyon was then carved by years of erosion and flash flooding as monsoon rainwater rushed through the narrow space, creating groovy grooves that are an art all their own.

**Antelope Canyon Navajo Tours.** As it is on Navajo land, Upper Antelope Canyon can only be visited on an official tour. There are several companies, but we booked through Antelope Canyon Navajo Tours and they were awesome. You'll meet at a group holding area and they shuttle you a few dusty miles to the canyon. Bring water! You'll need it and as of my visit they weren't selling any at the modest tour waiting area. Our Navajo guide, Mikea, was not only knowledgeable about the canyon's geology and history, but she also knew every camera angle and lighting trick. She rocked.

**Giddyup to Horseshoe Bend.** Just south of Page, Arizona is the incredible Horseshoe Bend. A horseshoe-shaped meander reveals the Colorado River far, far below. The cliffs are a thousand feet high and it's a total rush coming close to the edge. No doubt you've seen images of this place and wondered, "Where the heck is that??" It doesn't take too much imagination to see a grimacing face in the rock formation. It's a short 1.3 mile walk from the parking lot (right off US 89) to the observation deck. There's a small $10 fee but totally worth it. Bring water, it's hot and the sun is intense.

## AIRPLANE ROCK/CHAPEL CAVE, OHIO
### First-class hiking at Airplane Rock

Ohio's Hocking Hills region is packed with natural wonders — and packed with people trying to enjoy those natural wonders. But there are equally beautiful hikes without the crowds. Sometimes you gotta take the road (or trail) less traveled. Fortunately, you'll find friendly skies and first-class hiking at Airplane Rock.

The Airplane Rock Trail is a stunning path that's off the beaten path. This 4.5 mile loop trail is located near Rockbridge, Ohio, within the Hocking State Forest and not far from the far-more famous Conkles Hollow. The hiking trail runs on a bridle trail and riders get the right of way. It's listed on AllTrails as moderately challenging, but when it's muddy, which it often is, I'd say, "This one goes to 11." It's easy to lose a boot to the hungry mud.

While most people visit spring through fall, don't discount the beauty of a winter visit to Airplane Rock. The trails are far less busy (as in maybe NO ONE) and on a sunny day it's magical.

**Yes, it really looks like an airplane.** The challenging terrain leads you to a worthy reward: a magnificent rock outcropping shaped like the nose of an airplane. You'll need to peek at it from the side to realize the resemblance to an actual plane. But even if you don't, the airplane connection makes sense because when you stand on the overlook you'll feel like you're flying over the scenic Crane Hollow below. The panoramic views are breathtaking, especially at sunset.

*Pro tip:* If you want to see the sunset from here, you'll end up hiking back to the parking area in the dark forest. Time your departure wisely, and make sure your iPhone is charged and your flashlight app works. The walk back can be dangerous in the dark.

**Two natural wonders in one.** Another great benefit of this trail is that it's two natural wonders in one. Before or after Airplane Rock, be sure to visit Chapel Cave. Named for its cathedral-like appearance with a triangular opening and pointed top, this large recess cave is a hidden gem in the Hocking Forest. There's a little bit of Indiana Jones adventure waiting in there.

## SEVEN BRIDGES TRAIL, COLORADO
### "Raging Zen" in Colorado Springs

After moving my daughter Hannah to Colorado Springs, I was itching to hike some of the amazing trails there. And there are endless options. Having a few hours to myself while they unpacked, I borrowed her Jeep Wrangler and headed to the mountains.

One trail that caught my eye was the Seven Bridges Trail near Manitou Springs in North Cheyenne Cañon. It's a moderately-difficult 5.78 mile out-and-back and one of the area's most popular hikes. During its 1,597 ft. elevation gain, the trail follows a rushing stream that keeps it cool, even in the summer. From the parking lot you ascend the first half of the hike, and it can be challenging. Up, up, up. But all that elevation creates something spiritual and special: plenty of active waterfalls as the stream rushes downhill. I timed my hike just right, as it had rained heavily the night before, creating roaring rapids the entire way underneath those — you guessed it — seven bridges.

Hiking has always had a calming effect on me. I find my zen in nature. But there's an intoxicating contrast between a chill woods vibe and the adrenaline rush of rushing water. Seven Bridges delivered a frothy cocktail of contradictions that day, earning it the nickname Raging Zen.

## BLENDON WOODS, COLUMBUS
### Where I learned to woods walk

Blendon Woods Metro Park will always be a special place for me. This popular 653-acre park near Westerville is part of the wonderful Columbus and Franklin County Metro Park system, which provides natural green spaces and 230 miles of trails to central Ohio.

I grew up near there. I played frisbee golf after school there. I even had my first real teenage job there, working the long-gone Snack Shack with my best friend Greg. I'm pretty sure those two 16-year-old knuckleheads drove the head ranger boss to madness. Picture Wayne and Garth ineptly dishing up stale popcorn and melted slushies with a side order of Van Halen.

But most importantly, I began hiking there. As a kid with my parents, then as a teenager, and eventually with my own kids when they were young.

Blendon Woods features three short-ish loops totaling about five miles of trails. While most are ranked as easy, there are some decent elevation gains. The heavily forested trails are truly beautiful, with stream-cut ravines and exposed ripple rock sandstone. One of my favorite areas, near the dog park parking lot, features a pine forest section of trail. The path is carpeted with pine needles and when you're there a hush fills the air. Also worth noting are the meadow trails in the dog walking area that burst with bright wildflowers every spring.

Even though it's a suburban park and not very remote, there is a surprising abundance of wildlife. Especially around the 118-acre Walden Waterfowl Refuge and Thoreau Lake. It's a sanctuary for over 220 species of birds, including many songbirds, ducks, geese, herons, hawks and owls. Plus tons of frogs, toads, snakes (ugh), and more. Perhaps most famous of all is the flock of wild turkeys who call Blendon home. They often hang out in the parking lots, like rowdy teenagers looking for trouble.

CHAPTER 9

# Happy trails to you

*Your wellness is waiting*

With apologies to the one-of-a-kind Bob Ross, there's nothing like "The Joy of Panting."

The gasping for air, can't catch your breath, smiling from ear to ear exhilaration of reaching the top of a steep trail and appreciating that awe-inspiring view, as sweet oxygen returns you to normal. Yes, hiking can be breathtaking in more ways than one. Nature is a work of art, even if it *feels* like work sometimes. And despite that incline, and inclination to quit, we don't. We keep going. Because oddly enough, this thing makes us…happy.

Yes, those "happy little trees" and a happy little hike can be a powerful boost to your overall well-being. Slinging on that backpack, lacing up those boots, and hitting the trail offers a bundle of bubbly benefits.

DAVID HENTHORNE

## A WILD WORLD OF WELLNESS

Hiking is so much more than just a physical activity. That hiking trail is in fact a holistic path to wellness. From strengthening the body to inspiring the mind to healing the soul, the perks of a good woods walk are undeniable.

**A forest full of physical fitness.** As we've seen, the physical upside of hiking is undeniable. Our scientist friends say so. A good woods walk strengthens the cardiovascular system by increasing heart rate and improving blood flow. Our muscular endurance is enhanced as we navigate uneven terrain, climb inclines, and descend slopes. Hiking strengthens bones and improves joint health, especially as it helps us burn calories and build muscle mass. Regular hikes can even improve balance and coordination, reducing the risk of falls, particularly as we get older.

**Nature's stressbuster.** Studies show that spending time outdoors reduces stress and anxiety in big ways. In part because nature provides our busy minds a refuge from the constant barrage of stimuli in our daily lives. All those calls, emails, texts, tweets, traffic, and other worrisome interruptions. The forest fosters a state of blissful mindfulness. Immersing yourself in the relaxing sights, sounds, and smells of nature has a definite calming effect, lowering cortisol levels and promoting feelings of peace and, well... happiness. When we breathe in the fresh air and watch the sunlight dance on the trees, it's a natural mood enhancer. And speaking of sunlight, sun exposure during your hike provides a healthy dose of vitamin D, essential for mood regulation and overall well-being. Vitamin D deficiency has been linked to depression, so getting a sun-kissed dose on the trail can brighten your day, and your mood.

**A moving meditation.** Hiking gets your blood pumping and your body moving. This physical activity releases endorphins, those feel-good chemicals in your brain that create a natural sense of euphoria. Plus, the rhythmic motion of walking can be almost meditative, allowing you to clear your head and focus on the present moment. The gentle chirping of birds, rustling of leaves, and gurgling of a babbling brook can lull the mind into a state of present-moment awareness, allowing negative thoughts and anxieties to just fade away.

**A sense of accomplishment.** Reaching the top of a challenging climb or completing a longer trail provides a satisfying sense of get 'er done. It's a reminder of your own strength and perseverance, boosting your confidence and self-esteem. This can be particularly beneficial for those struggling with low self-esteem, depression, or facing personal challenges. Finishing a tough trail can translate into a renewed belief in your ability to overcome obstacles in other areas of life. And how's this for taking on a new challenge: Hiking can even inspire you to become more environmentally conscious, willing to protect these natural spaces and trails that give us so much.

**Connecting with yourself (and maybe others).** Hiking allows you to disconnect from the constant buzz of technology and reconnect with yourself. It's a chance to reflect, be present, and appreciate the beauty that surrounds you. This mind-body harmony is essential for overall well-being. Hiking with friends or family adds an important social element, fostering connection and shared experiences.

> Some of my greatest hiking experiences have been on international group hiking trips where not only do you get to explore great new destinations, but you get to spend many hours getting to know people from all over the world. Listening to views from around the globe makes you realize how small the world is and how humans from every country all aspire to the same goals in life: family, love of others, and peace. **– Scott, Colorado**

# WELLNESS IN THE WOODS

My three favorite things about hiking: Peace, Nature, Mindfulness.  **– Carie, Ohio**

I am thankful for living where I am to experience nature through trails. Whenever I travel I try to hike. It's a fantastic way to experience something new and to meet people along the way.  **– John, Oregon**

Once while hiking in southern Ohio, I had a mystical reckoning with a hummingbird who had likely mistaken my daypack as a flower. He buzzed around me for about 15 minutes. We were high up on a bluff and I felt like he certainly had something to say if only I knew his language. Perhaps "Show me the nectar!"
**– Lisa, Ohio**

To me an ideal hike is about challenge level, and witnessing something new and unexpected. One time I was on a 6-mile muddy, roller-coaster-of-a-trail hike and heard a tree fall. I will never forget the sound. That hike was perfect.  **– Hannah, Colorado**

DAVID HENTHORNE

**MAKE HIKING YOUR HAPPY PLACE**

So, can hiking actually make you happy? Can it put you on a better path, help your health, and cure what ails you? Throughout these pages we've seen that scientists think it can. It sure seems that America's 60 million hiking fanatics think so too.

And so do I.

Here's a final happy thought. Most hiking trails have "blazes" to mark the route. They're color-coded circles to keep you on the right path. If you're on the red trail, you'll see red markers on trees every 50 feet or so. If you're trekking the blue trail, you'll see blue blazes. It's especially helpful when trails intersect or split off or it's a confusing mishmash of vegetation. Sometimes in the middle of a long hike, when the zen kicks in, I imagine each of those circular blazes is actually a happy smiley face grinning back at me. Encouraging and urging me forward, on the trail and in life.

WELLNESS IN THE WOODS

## "OF ALL THE PATHS YOU TAKE IN LIFE, MAKE SURE A FEW OF THEM ARE DIRT."

— JOHN MUIR

# Acknowledgements

Thank you to those who inspired me to get up, get out there, and get to writing this book.

Thank you to my family, especially my parents Harry and Carolyn for giving me a loving zest for life, an appreciation for the little things, and a natural curiosity about the world. I hope you are up there right now squabbling over Scrabble and cutting a rug on heaven's dance floor.

Thank you to my adventure-loving, wilderness-running, always smiling, Rocky Mountain-highing daughter Hannah. No matter the weather on the trail, your sunny disposition always shines through. Keep on Happying, Birdie Girl. And special thanks for the stunning photo on this book's cover.

Thanks to my blooming botanist son Dylan, for his unwavering passion for every kind of plant and commitment to a vegan lifestyle. A woods walk with him often turns into a "what's that one?" quiz show as you point to a plant and he invariably knows the answer. You've taught me more than you know and never cease to amaze me.

Thanks to my other nurturing family, the one I've worked with for over 30 years. The talented team at Ron Foth Advertising has become much more than friends as we've traveled the world and made marketing magic.

And thank you to my life-changing partner Carie. How did I ever find the one person on Earth who loves hiking as much as I do? Looking forward to exploring more trails and more life with you. I'm happy my hiking boots are right beside yours.

# About the author

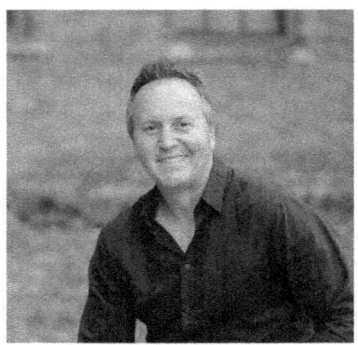

**David Henthorne** is an award-winning creative director, writer, and Certified Tourism Ambassador. He has created ad campaigns for many of America's top brands, been a speaker at national travel conferences, and is a board trustee for the Ohio State Parks Foundation. When he's not making ads that stick in your head, he's probably hiking or thinking about hiking. He shares his adventures at his website, WorldOfWanders.com.

# WELLNESS IN THE WOODS

www.ingramcontent.com/pod-product-compliance
Lightning Source LLC
Chambersburg PA
CBHW020547030426
42337CB00013B/996